D1798452

RECENT DEVELOPMENTS IN THE STUDY OF

Benign
Breast Disease

RECENT DEVELOPMENTS IN THE STUDY OF

Benign
Breast Disease

The Proceedings of the
4th International Benign Breast Symposium, Manchester, April 1991

Edited by R. E. Mansel

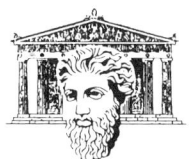

The Parthenon Publishing Group
International Publishers in Medicine, Science & Technology

Casterton Hall, Carnforth,
Lancs, LA6 2LA, UK

120 Mill Road, Park Ridge,
New Jersey 07656, USA

Published in the UK by
The Parthenon Publishing Group Limited
Casterton Hall, Carnforth,
Lancs. LA6 2LA, England

Published in the USA by
The Parthenon Publishing Group Inc.
120 Mill Road,
Park Ridge,
New Jersey, 07656, USA

British Library Cataloguing-in-Publication Data
International Benign Breast Disease Symposium
(4th 1991 Manchester)
  Benign breast disease.
  I. Title   II. Mansel, R.E.
  618.1

  ISBN 1-85070-386-8

Library of Congress Cataloging-in-Publication Data
International Benign Breast Symposium (4th: 1991: Manchester, England)
  Benign Breast disease: the proceedings of the 4th International Benign Breast
Symposium, Manchester, April 1991/edited by R.E. Mansel.
    p. cm.
  Includes bibliographical references and index.
  ISBN 1-85070-386-8
    1. Breast—Diseases—Congresses. I. Mansel, R. E.   II. Title.
    [DNLM: 1. Breast Diseases—congresses. WP 840 I595b 1991]
RG491.I58 1991
618.1'9—dc20
DNLM/DLC
for Library of Congress   91-37361
                                                                          CIP

Phototypesetting by Lasertext Ltd., Manchester
Printed and bound in Great Britain by
Redwood Press Ltd., Melksham, Wiltshire

Contents

Contents

List of principal contributors

E. Alvarez Gardiol
Centro de Mastología
Dorrego 548
2000 Rosario
Argentina

S. Battersby
Department of Pathology
University of Edinburgh
Medical School
Teviot Place
Edinburgh EH8 9AG
UK

N.F. Boyd
Division of Epidemiology and
    Statistics
Ontario Cancer Institute
500 Sherbourne Street
Toronto M4X 1K9
Canada

U. Chetty
University Department of Surgery
The Royal Infirmary
Edinburgh EH3 9YW
UK

I.D. Campbell
University Surgical Unit
Southampton General Hospital
Southampton SO9 4XY
UK

J.M. Dixon
University Department of Surgery
The Royal Infirmary
Edinburgh EH3 9YW
UK

M. Elstein
Department of Obstetrics and
    Gynaecology
Withington Hospital
Manchester
UK

I.S. Fentiman
ICRF Clinical Oncology Unit
Guy's Hospital
London SE1 9RT
UK

M.H. Galea
Department of Surgery
Nottingham City Hospital
Hucknall Road
Nottingham NG5 1PB
UK

C.A. Gateley
University Hospital of South
    Manchester
Nell Lane
West Didsbury
Manchester M20 8LR
UK

P.B. Guyer
Southampton & Salisbury Breast
  Screening Unit
RSH Hospital
Southampton SO9 4PE
UK

H. Hamed
ICRF Clinical Oncology Unit
Guy's Hospital
London SE1 9RT
UK

K. Horgan
University Department of Surgery
University Hospital of Wales
Heath Park
Cardiff CF4 4XN
UK

L.E. Hughes
University Department of Surgery
University Hospital of Wales
Heath Park
Cardiff CF4 4XN
UK

I.J. Laidlaw
University Hospital of South
  Manchester
Nell Lane
West Didsbury
Manchester M20 8LR
UK

S.J. Leinster
Royal Liverpool Hospital
Prescot Road
Liverpool L7 8XP
UK

K. McPherson
London School of Hygiene &
  Tropical Medicine
University of London
Keppel Street
London WC1E 7HT
UK

P.R. Maddox
University Department of Surgery
University Hospital of Wales
Heath Park
Cardiff CF4 4XN
UK

R.E. Mansel
Department of Surgery
University Hospital of South
  Manchester
Nell Lane
West Didsbury
Manchester M20 8LR
UK

M.E. Miers
University Department of Surgery
University Hospital of Wales
Heath Park
Cardiff CF4 4XN
UK

W.R. Miller
Imperial Cancer Research Fund
Medical Oncology Unit
Western General Hospital
Edinburgh EH4 2XU
UK

List of principal contributors

I.J. Monypenny
Department of Surgery
Llandough Hospital
Penarth
South Glamorgan
UK

M.C. Nicolson
Royal Marsden Hospital
Downs Road
Sutton
Surrey SM2 5PT
UK

A.M. Schor
CRC Department of Medical
    Oncology
Christie Hospital NHS Trust
Wilmslow Road
Manchester M20 9BX
UK

N. Tomimatsu
Kanazawa University of Medicine
Department of Obstetrics and
    Gynecology
13-1 Takaramachi
Kanazawa 920
Japan

R.A. Walker
Department of Pathology
Clinical Sciences Building
Leicester Royal Infirmary
PO Box 65
Leicester LE2 7LX
UK

Foreword

It is my pleasure to write the Foreword to this volume reporting the papers presented at the 4th International Benign Breast Symposium in Manchester, April 11-12, 1991. These meetings began in Cardiff over 10 years ago and have increased in popularity over the years, with this year's meeting welcoming delegates and speakers from Japan, Argentina and Italy from the audience. The original aim of the Symposium was to give a comprehensive review of the clinical management of benign breast diseases suitable for the interested clinician and to cover some of the relevant research areas. The meetings have continued with the aim of being educational with expert reviews on common conditions mixed in with good basic science.

In the 1991 meeting, several papers looked at the management of breast pain, and the technical aspects of cytology and needle localization biopsy were reviewed in the 'How I do it' session. The management of problem conditions such as the recurrent duct fistula and the benign pathology of screening were covered. A whole session was devoted to the highly topical subject of chemoprevention of breast cancer and measurement of risk factors for cancer. These studies are at the forefront of current clinical research, as is shown by the expansion of the Marsden Tamoxifen Prevention Trial into several other centres. An excellent review of the epidemiology of hormones and cancer risk was given by Professor Klim McPherson, with the clarity and authority one expects from a protegé of the Oxford Epidemiology School.

The basic science session concentrated on the very exciting work now proceeding in the area of epithelial–stromal relationships, and it is clear that these fundamental studies hold out the prospect of translation into practical clinical therapies in the not-too-distant future.

The meeting was thoroughly enjoyed by all and the Symposium dinner held in Manchester's China town was a memorable feast. I wish to record my thanks to all the delegates and the speakers for being so prompt in the production of their manuscripts to allow early publication. My thanks also go to Sterling Winthrop for an educational grant in support of the meeting. I look forward to seeing you all again in Manchester in 1993.

R.E. Mansel

SECTION 1

Mastalgia

I

The Cardiff Mastalgia Clinic experience of the natural history of mastalgia

C.A. Gateley, M. Miers, J.F. Skone and R.E. Mansel

INTRODUCTION

Breast pain or mastalgia is a common condition which is reported by over half the female population if questioned directly[1], and accounts for 45–50% of presentations to breast clinics[1]. An understanding of the natural history of mastalgia is required to enable the clinician to counsel the patient adequately, and to help in deciding whether to prescribe drug treatment.

A dedicated mastalgia clinic was established within the Department of Surgery at the Welsh National School of Medicine in 1973. Patients are only referred from the breast clinic if the pain continues to be severe after exclusion of overt pathology, and reassurance. On referral to the mastalgia clinic the pain is classified into cyclical and non-cyclical mastalgia[2], and the severity measured using a breast pain chart[3]. This clinic reported in 1983 on the natural history of breast pain, 2–7 years after initial assessment[4]. We have updated this study to provide at least 10 years' follow-up of the patients.

METHODS

Postal questionnaires were sent to 235 patients with cyclical and non-cyclical mastalgia who had previously been studied in 1983. Five patients who were known to have developed breast cancer and one who was treated by subcutaneous mastectomy for mastalgia were not followed-up in this way. Altogether, 183 questionnaires were returned (eight uncompleted) and a further 24 replies were obtained by telephone or personal interview.

The questionnaire asked if the breast pain had continued or resolved. If the pain had continued, its present classification and severity was determined or, if resolution had occurred, with what this was associated. Duration of the pain was calculated from onset to follow-up if still present, or from onset to resolution.

RESULTS

A total of 199 (85%) usable replies were obtained, 139 from patients who had initially been classified to have cyclical mastalgia, and 60 from patients with non-cyclical mastalgia.

Cyclical mastalgia

Pain continued in 82 patients (59%), with a mean duration of 15 years (range, 10–38 years), though 40 patients felt that the pain was now less severe and only 14 felt that it was worse. In 30 patients the pain remained obviously cyclical in nature, but in 34 women the nature of the pain had changed to non-cyclical and, in four patients, to continuous pain. The remaining 14 were unable to classify the pain, mainly because of having had a hysterectomy.

Pain had resolved in 57 (41%), after a mean duration of 9 years (range, 6 months to 30 years), and in 49 patients resolution was associated with an hormonal event (Table 1).

Non-cyclical mastalgia

Pain continued in 35 patients (58%), with a mean duration of 15 years (range, 10–34 years), though 13 patients felt that the pain was now less severe and only four felt that it was worse. In 28 patients the pain remained non-cyclical in nature; two patients felt that the nature of the

Table 1   Events associated with breast pain resolution. (Number of occurrences, followed by percentage in brackets)

Event	Cyclical mastalgia ($n = 57$)	Non-cyclical mastalgia ($n = 25$)
Pregnancy/lactation	10 (18)	1 (4)
Contraceptive pill	3 (5)	—
Menopause	29 (51)	9 (36)
Hysterectomy	3 (5)	—
Hysterectomy and oophorectomy	4 (7)	1 (4)
Spontaneous	2 (4)	8 (32)
Other	6	6

pain had changed to cyclical; in three women the pain was continuous, and only two were unable to classify the pain because of having had a hysterectomy.

Pain had resolved in 25 patients (42%), after a mean duration of 7 years (range, 4 months to 19 years). In 11 women resolution was associated with an hormonal event and spontaneous resolution occurred in eight patients (Table 1).

DISCUSSION

This 10-year review confirms the chronic nature of severe cyclical and non-cyclical mastalgia, the majority of women having symptoms for at least 5 years. Where pain continues the classification may change with time, as more than half of the patients initially classified as cyclical now have non-cyclical mastalgia. Cyclical mastalgia always resolves at the menopause, but in these patients whose pain has changed nature, the menopause may have no effect on severity. It is less common for the nature of the pain to become cyclical in patients initially classified to have non-cyclical mastalgia. This may be related to patients with non-cyclical mastalgia being older at presentation[2], or may indicate that the natural evolution is from cyclical to non-cyclical mastalgia after a number of years.

Resolution of cyclical mastalgia is normally associated with hormonal events such as the menopause and spontaneous resolution is rare. However, in non-cyclical mastalgia, spontaneous resolution is as common as hormonally related resolution. Studies of non-cyclical mastalgia have shown lesser abnormalities of hormone release[5] and a lesser response to drug treatment[6]. A recent reassessment of patients with non-cyclical mastalgia has suggested that when chest wall pain is excluded by careful examination, the response to drug treatment in true non-cyclical mastalgia approaches that expected in cyclical mastalgia[7]. The increased proportion of patients with non-cyclical mastalgia who experienced a menopause-associated resolution, 36% in this study compared with 19% in the earlier[4], suggests an underlying endocrine abnormality in these patients.

Cyclical and non-cyclical mastalgia both run a chronic relapsing course. If mastalgia is severe and developed at a young age, the pain is likely to persist for many years and repeated courses of drug treatment are likely. This has important implications as long-term treatment for mastalgia may be needed, usually on an intermittent basis although continuous low-dose regimens may also be suitable[8]. If pain develops shortly before the menopause, treatment may be delayed in the knowledge that resolution will occur in patients with cyclical mastalgia and in some patients with non-cyclical mastalgia.

ACKNOWLEDGEMENT

We thank Mrs D. Skone for her painstaking work in the collation of the data.

REFERENCES

1. Hughes, L.E., Mansel, R.E. and Webster, D.J.T. (1989). *Benign Disorders and Diseases of the Breast*, pp. 75–92. (London: Baillière Tindall)
2. Preece, P.E., Hughes, L.E., Mansel, R.E., Baum, M., Bolton, P.M. and Gravelle, I.H. (1976). Clinical symptoms of mastalgia. *Lancet*, **2**, 670–3
3. Maddox, P.R. and Mansel, R.E. (1989). Management of breast pain and nodularity. *World J. Surg.*, **13**, 699–705
4. Wiseby, J.R., Kumar, S., Mansel, R.E., Preece, P.E., Pye, J.K. and Hughes, L.E. (1983). Natural history of breast pain. *Lancet*, **2**, 672–4
5. Kumar, S., Mansel, R.E., Hughes, L.E., Woodhead, J.S., Edwards, C.A., Scanton, M.F. and Newcombe, R.G. (1984). Prolactin response to thyrotro-

pin-releasing hormone stimulation and dopaminergic inhibition in benign breast disease. *Cancer*, **53**, 1311–5

6. Pye, J.K., Mansel, R.E. and Hughes, L.E. (1985). Clinical experience of drug treatments for mastalgia. *Lancet*, **2**, 373–6

7. Maddox, P.R., Harrison, B.J., Mansel, R.E. and Hughes, L.E. (1989). Non-cyclical mastalgia: an improved classification and treatment. *Br. J. Surg.*, **76**, 901–4

8. Harrison, B.J., Maddox, P.R. and Mansel, R.E. (1989). Maintenance therapy of cyclical mastalgia using low-dose danazol. *J.R. Coll. Surg. Edinb.*, **34**, 79–81

2

Experiences with tamoxifen and goserelin in women with mastalgia

I.S. Fentiman, H. Hamed and M. Caleffi

BACKGROUND

Although the Breast Clinic at Guy's Hospital was originally set up by Sir Hedley Atkins to treat 'mastitis', its work had been devoted largely to the management of malignant disease. By 1984, it was apparent that much of the clinical workload comprised women with mastalgia. Although the majority of such individuals required no treatment other than reassurance, there were a few in whom the breast pain was having a major impact on their life. At that time the main drugs in use were bromocriptine and danazol, both of which were sometimes associated with intolerable side-effects at the dosages recommended. There was some anecdotal evidence that the agent tamoxifen, deemed to be an antioestrogen, could relieve the symptoms of mastalgia. This was supported by use in a few patients at Guy's and so it was felt to be appropriate to conduct a prospective randomized clinical trial.

THE TAMOXIFEN TRIALS

The first study was of double-blind, placebo-controlled, cross-over design[1]. Eligible patients had self-rated moderate/severe mastalgia which had been present for a minimum of 6 months. None had received any endocrine therapy for at least 3 months before entry. All completed pain analogue cards for 2 months before entry. They were then allocated at random to receive either tamoxifen 20 mg daily or placebo (vitamin C, 50 mg daily) for 3 months. Those who failed to respond were switched to the alternative treatment arm. A total of 60 patients were entered into the trial.

Success, as measured by a 50% reduction in mean pain score was achieved in 22 (71%) of those given tamoxifen and 11 (38%) of the placebo group. Of the 18 placebo-treated patients who did not respond, 12 were given tamoxifen and pain relief occurred in eight (75%). Side-effects were reported by 26% of the tamoxifen group and 10% of the placebo group, the commonest complaints being hot flushes and increased vaginal discharge.

After stopping treatment, symptoms relapsed in approximately 50% of cases. In an attempt to reduce both the relapse rate and the incidence of side-effects, a second trial was conducted to examine both dosage and duration of treatment with tamoxifen. Another 60 patients, with similar eligibility criteria to those in the first trial, were randomized within a factorial 2 × 2 design study[2]. They received tamoxifen at a dosage of either 10 mg or 20 mg for either 3 or 6 months.

Among patients given tamoxifen at 10 mg the response rate was 26 out of 29 (90%) compared with 24 out of 28 (86%) in those receiving 20 mg daily. Thus reduction of dosage did not result in loss of efficacy, although side-effects were reduced significantly in those given 10 mg, being 21% compared with 64% in the higher dosage group. Prolongation of treatment from 3 to 6 months did not affect response rate, nor the relapse rate.

Thus the two trials demonstrated the efficacy and lack of serious short-term toxicity of tamoxifen. Nevertheless, there were worries about the effect of long-term tamoxifen administration to women with benign conditions because of reported cataracts and hepatocellular carcinomas in rats given very high dosages, despite no comparable data being reported for humans[3]. Another problem was the high relapse rate and it was hypothesized that a more substantial endocrine alteration might be needed to achieve long-term control of severe cyclical mastalgia. Such a possibility emerged in the form of the luteinizing hormone releasing hormone (LHRH) agonist, goserelin.

THE GOSERELIN TRIAL

This was conducted as a non-randomized study, in order to gain maximum information on both efficacy and side-effects. Initially, 21 women with refractory or recurrent moderate/severe mastalgia were given goserelin at a dosage of 3.6 mg subcutaneously every 4 weeks for a total of six implants[4]. Originally local anaesthesia was used before giving the implant but soon it was found that this was unnecessary. The study was extended with a further 33 patients, including 16 patients with previously untreated mastalgia.

A simplified pain scoring system was used, with a square for each day. Patients were asked to fill in the square if the pain was severe, half fill it if pain was less severe and mark a central dot if no pain was present. As a score, 2 points were given for a full square, 1 for half a square and 0 for a dotted square. The pretreatment score was the sum of the values for the 28 days prior to the first implant and successful pain relief was defined as a 50% reduction in the mean score over the 28 days following each implant.

A total of 31 (57%) of patients had cyclical pain and in 23 (43%) the mastalgia was non-cyclical. The overall response rate was 46 out of 54 (85%) as shown in Table 1. One patient dropped out after the first implant. Almost all the women with cyclical pain responded to treatment but more than 50% took more than 1 month to respond. Thus it would not be of value to use a goserelin implant as a therapeutic test, although it was an effective treatment, and those who failed to respond were resistant to all other therapies. It is of interest that an eventual response occurred in 70% of those with non-cyclical mastalgia. The major problem was the high incidence of side-effects reported by almost all patients including hot flushes (87%), headache (57%), diminished libido (37%), nausea/vomiting (28%) and depression/irritability (24%). A total

Table 1   Response to goserelin treatment

	Cyclical pain	Non-cyclical pain
Patients	31	23
Success	30 (97%)	16 (70%)
Time to response		
1 month	13	2
> 1 month	17	14

of 11 patients (20%) failed to complete the course of six injections. The relapse rate after stopping goserelin was 80%, with a mean follow-up of 6 months.

FUTURE WORK

The results of the goserelin study suggest that this agent will not be useful for the majority of patients with mastalgia because of the high incidence of side-effects, together with the high relapse rate after cessation of treatment. It would appear that long-term therapy is needed for many patients with mastalgia and this has to be as non-toxic as possible. The study which is planned will give 3 months of tamoxifen at a dosage of 10 mg daily. Among those who respond there will be a 3-way randomization: one group will continue with tamoxifen, 10 mg daily; another will be treated with evening primrose oil, and another group will receive a placebo. It is possible that a combined approach, inducing remission with tamoxifen, and then attempting maintenance treatment with evening primrose oil might prove to be an effective approach.

REFERENCES

1. Fentiman, I.S., Caleffi, M., Brame, K., Chaudary, M.A. and Hayward, J.L. (1986). Double blind controlled trial of tamoxifen therapy for mastalgia. *Lancet*, **1**, 287–8
2. Fentiman, I.S., Caleffi, M., Hamed, H. and Chaudary, M.A. (1988). Dosage and duration of tamoxifen treatment for mastalgia: a randomised trial. *Br. J. Surg.*, **75**, 845–8
3. Fentiman, I.S. and Powles, T.J. (1987). Tamoxifen and benign breast conditions. *Lancet*, **2**, 1070–1
4. Hamed, H., Chaudary, M.A., Caleffi, M. and Fentiman, I.S. (1990). LHRH analogue for treatment of recurrent and refractory mastalgia. *Ann. R. Coll. Surg. Eng.*, **72**, 221–4

3

Ultrasonic changes of mastopathy associated with danazol

S. Terada, N. Tomimatsu, N. Suzuki, T. Kohama, K. Akasofu and E. Nishida

Benign breast disease can often be seen in women whose endocrinological milieu is in imbalance. Benign breast disease shows complicated histological lesions, including proliferation of mammary epithelial cells, cystic formation and fibrosis. In Japan there are less patients with breast cancer than in other countries, especially USA and Europe, although recently there have been reports on the increase of cases of breast cancer corresponding with the dietary increase in fat-rich food. As a consequence, Japanese researchers have paid little attention until now to benign breast disease. However for the first time in Japan, we have recently reported findings in the treatment of benign breast disease which occurred concurrently in patients who had endometriosis and who were treated with danazol[1].

MATERIAL AND METHODS

A total of 20 patients with benign disease (mastopathy and fibrocystic disease) and with concurrent endometriosis were admitted to the present study for 2 years. Their ages ranged from 28 to 48 years, with a mean age of 40.4 years.

The criteria for diagnosis of benign breast disease were:

(1) Breast pain and/or tenderness sustained for more than 3 months cyclically;

(2) Palpation of breast masses showing ill-defined, elastic and coarse granular masses;

(3) Many microcystic, spotted and linear echos were found in the mammary glands under ultrasonographic examination;

(4) Radiographic findings were like ground-glass and there was homogeneous shadow.

(5) In the cases with nipple discharge, foam cells and/or apocrine cells were found cytologically.

Danazol was administered to the patients in a regimen of 300 mg/day for a duration of 3–6 months. Blood tests were performed (blood cell counts, liver function test, etc.) and changes in breast pain, tenderness and nipple discharge were measured once a month. Palpation of the breasts and ultrasonographic examination were carried out monthly. Degrees of pain, tenderness, nodularity and ultrasonographic findings of fibroglandular tissues were judged in terms of a classification, modified from Humphrey and Estes's classification[2]. Table 1 shows this classification of disease severity. Each factor is composed of four grades.

RESULTS

Table 2 shows the therapeutic effects of danazol for benign breast disease.

As an example, consider case 5, a 38-year-old patient. A pretreatment ultrasonograph shows a microcystic, spotted and linear echo in the rich mammary parenchyma (Figure 1). A pretreatment radiograph shows a ground-glass-like shadow (Figure 2). After 3 months' treatment with danazol the ultrasonograph shows that lesions seen before treatment have disappeared and mammary parenchyma have decreased (Figure 3).

Softening and reduction of indurations and lumps in terms of the ultrasonographic findings imply that the proliferation of glandular components in the glandular parenchyma was decreased as a result of danazol administration.

Table I   Classification of disease severity (modified from Humphrey and Estes[2])

(1)	Pain	
	none	1
	mild	2
	moderate	3
	severe	4
(2)	Tenderness	
	none	1
	mild	2
	moderate	3
	severe	4
(3)	Nodularity (presence of nodules)	
	none	1
	single	2
	few	3
	numerous	4
(4)	Areas of fibroglandular tissue (ultrasound)	
	sparse	1
	moderate	2
	prominent localized	3
	massive diffuse spread	4

Effects of danazol on pain

Breast pain disappeared in 15 patients and the pain was alleviated in the other five patients. An improvement in symptoms was measured in all patients, with the mean score decreasing from 2.95 to 1.25.

Effects of danazol on tenderness

After 3 months of danazol treatment, tenderness disappeared in seven patients and alleviation of tenderness was found in the remaining 13 patients, with the mean score decreasing from 2.95 to 1.65.

Effects of danazol on nodularity

Glandular nodules were reduced in 15 patients and no changes were found in five patients. The hardness of nodules was decreased in all patients, with a mean score falling from 3.2 to 2.4.

Table 2 Therapeutic effects of danazol for benign breast disease (mastopathy)

Cases	Age (years)	Pain Before	Pain After	Tenderness Before	Tenderness After	Nodularity Before	Nodularity After	Areas of lesion (ultrasound) Before	Areas of lesion (ultrasound) After
1	37	3	2	3	2	4	3	4	2
2	34	3	1	3	1	3	2	3	2
3	38	3	2	3	2	4	3	4	2
4	48	3	1	3	1	3	2	2	1
5	38	3	1	3	2	4	3	4	2
6	46	3	1	3	2	3	2	3	2
7	40	3	2	3	2	3	3	3	2
8	46	2	1	2	1	2	1	2	1
9	44	3	1	3	2	3	2	3	2
10	45	3	1	3	2	3	2	3	2
11	40	3	1	3	2	3	3	3	2
12	37	3	1	3	2	3	2	3	2
13	35	3	1	3	1	3	3	3	2
14	44	3	1	3	1	3	2	3	2
15	43	3	1	3	2	4	3	4	2
16	47	3	2	3	2	4	3	4	2
17	44	3	1	3	1	3	1	2	1
18	36	3	1	3	1	3	3	2	1
19	28	3	1	3	2	2	2	3	2
20	32	3	1	3	2	4	3	4	2
(Mean ± SD)	40.4 ± 5.44	2.95 ± 0.22	1.25 ± 0.44	2.95 ± 0.22	1.65 ± 0.48	3.2 ± 0.61	2.4 ± 0.68	3.1 ± 0.71	1.8 ± 0.41

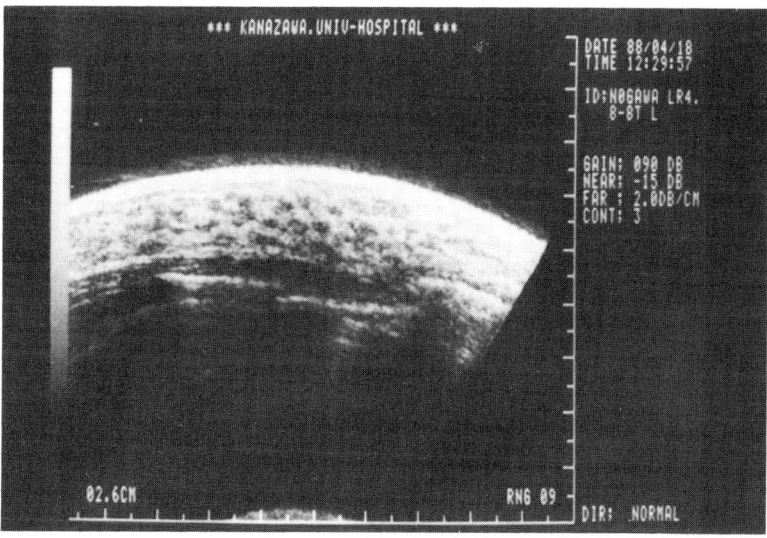

Figure 1 Breast ultrasonagraph of Case 5, before treatment, showing microcystic, spotted and linear echos in the rich mammary parenchyma

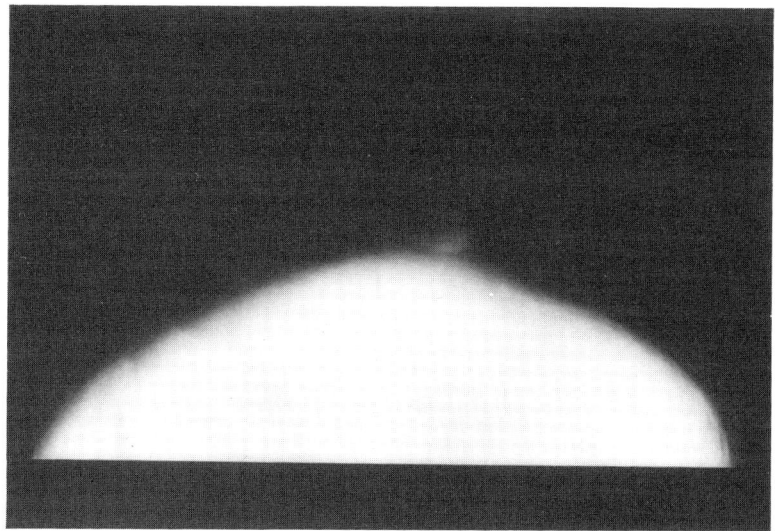

Figure 2 Mammogram of Case 5, before treatment, showing a ground-glass-like shadow

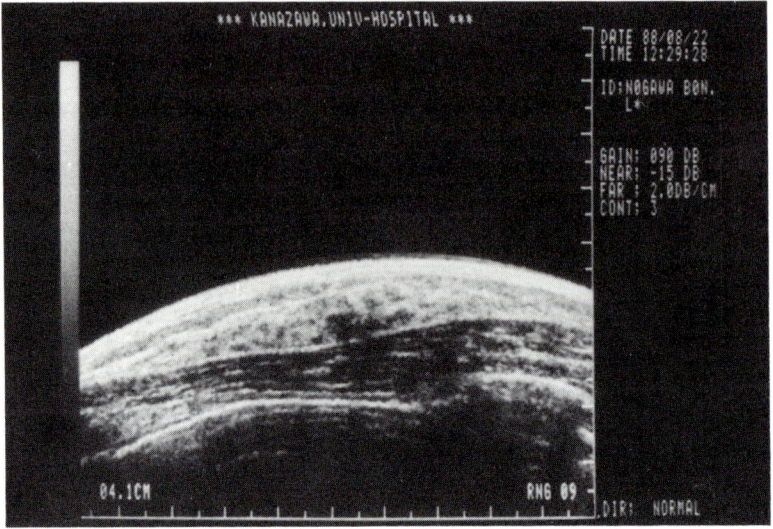

Figure 3 Breast ultrasonograph of Case 5 after 3 months' treatment with danazol. Lesions disappeared and mammary parenchyma have decreased

Effects on areas of fibroglandular tissue

The volume of glandular nodules was reduced as measured on ultrasonographic examination. The average score was lowered to 1.80 from a pretreatment score of 3.10.

DISCUSSION

Mastopathy is one of the most common diseases among mature women. Patients with this disease, with a noticeable breast mass, complain of cyclic breast pain and tenderness. The pain increases during luteal phases and diminishes during menstrual phases. These symptoms are known to disappear during pregnancy and lactating periods. It has been pointed out that cases with mastopathy are complicated with luteal insufficiency or insufficiency of prolactin secretion. It is important to realize that abnormalities in the endocrinological milieu cause this disease, particularly an absolute or relative excess of oestrogen[3].

Therapies for mastopathy consist of the administration of antioestrogen, for example dromostanorone, epithiostanol and tamoxifen[4]. In Japan, danazol is used for endometriosis but not for mastopathy.

The pharmacological effects of danazol are firstly, prevention of the midcycle surge of luteinizing hormone and follicle stimulating hormone, secondly, suppression of prolactin secretion, thirdly, direct suppression of oestrogen production in the ovary, fourthly, combination of the androgen and progesterone receptors, and finally, blocking of the oestrogen receptor[5]. Danazol is claimed to be useful for treating mastopathy due to the latter four effects. We used to encounter breast atrophy as a side-effect of danazol treatment of endometriosis. More recently, Mansel *et al.*[6] reported that treatment with danazol was effective for mastopathy.

The regimen of danazol for mastopathy used elsewhere is normally 200–400 mg per day for 3–6 months in other countries[7,8]; we tested, for the first time in Japan, treatments of 300 mg per day for 3–6 months.

The effectiveness of drug treatments for mastopathy is judged according to the reduction of symptoms, namely the alleviation or disappearance of pain and tenderness, and the softening or reduction of nodularity. Radiographic diagnostic methods for mastopathy are mammography and xeromammography, but methods involving frequent radiographic exposure are harmful to the patient. In contrast, ultrasonographic examination is harmless and can be carried out frequently[9].

Mastopathy histologically shows the proliferation and retardation of mammary epithelium and stroma[10]. It is said to be impossible to detect changes in mammary parenchyma, except by histological methods. But ultrasonography can distinguish mammary epithelial proliferation as low-echo areas and mammary stroma as high-echo areas[9]. Because of this, we consider that ultrasonographic examination permits the quantitative and qualitative changes in the mammary parenchyma to be followed, in cases of mastopathy.

In this study, the mean age of cases was 40.4 ± 5.4 years and this coincides with that of the former report.

It was concluded that danazol treatments of 300 mg per day for 3–6 months were effective treatments for mastopathy, in agreement with earlier reports from other countries.

REFERENCES

1. Terada, S., Tomimatsu, N., Suzuki, N., Kohama, T. and Akasofu, K. (1991). Clinical investigation of danazol therapy for mastopathy. *Sanfujinka no sekai*, **43**, 55–9

2. Humphrey, L.J. and Estes, N.C. (1979). Aspects of fibrocystic disease of the breast. Treatment with danazol. *Postgrad. Med. J.*, **55**, 48–51

3. Melis, G.B., Guarnini, G., Paoletti, A.M., Petacchi, F.D., Ricci, G., Strigini, F. and Selli, M. (1983). Clinical significance of hormonal evaluation in peripheral blood and breast cyst fluid of women with benign breast disease. In Angeli, A., Bradlow, H.L. and Dogliotti, L. (eds.) *Endocrinology of Cystic Breast Disease*, pp. 101–12. (New York: Raven Press)

4. Fournier, D., Junkermann, H., Stolz, W., Weber, E., Krapfe, E. and Fersizoglou, N. (1989). Hormonal and non-hormonal medical therapy of benign breast disease. *Horm. Res.*, **32**, 28–31

5. Rannevik, G. and Thorell, J.I. (1984). The influence of danazol on pituitary function and on the ovarian follicular hormone secretion in premenopausal women. *Acta Obstet. Gynecol. Scand.*, **123**, 89–94

6. Mansel, R.E. (1985). A double-blind trial of danazol in benign breast disease. *J.R. Soc. Med.*, **76**, 89–94

7. Locker, A.P., Hinton, C.P., Roebuck, E.J. and Blamey, R.W. (1989). Long-term follow up of patients treated with a single course of danazol for recurrent breast cysts. *Br. J. Pract., Symp. Suppl.*, **68**, 100–1

8. Andrews, W.C. (1990). Hormonal management of fibrocystic disease of the breast. *J. Reprod. Med.*, **35**, 87–90

9. Wood, C.B., Tsikos, C., Keane, P. and Yung, E. (1989). Ultrasound assessment response to therapy of clinically undetected breast cysts. *Br. J. Clin. Pract., Symp. Suppl.*, **68**, 102

10. Greenblatt, R.B., Chaddha, J.S., Teran, A.Z. and Lewis, A. (1984). Fibrocystic breast disease: pathophysiology, hormonology, treatment. *Contemp. Surg.*, **24**, 49–60

4

The Manchester Restandol trial

*I.J. Laidlaw, C. Gateley, P. Gray, J. Russell, R.E. Mansel and
A.W.M.C. Owen*

INTRODUCTION

Approximately 16% of women seek advice about benign disorders of
the breast during their lifetime[1]. A quarter of new referrals to a breast
clinic are for pain[2] and in about 10% of women symptoms are sufficient
to interfere with their normal daily routine. Important causes of breast
pain such as carcinoma, cyst and abscess should be treated on their
merits. The remainder may be classified into three main groups: cyclical,
non-cyclical and miscellaneous causes[3]. Despite the lack of consistent
histological or endocrinological abnormalities within groups, this classification is useful because of predictable response to certain drugs.
Reviews of the aetiology of cyclical breast pain have concluded that a
hormonal cause was most likely, although proof was inconclusive[3,4].
Various measures of androgen status have been found to be either
elevated, depressed or normal in many trials[4]. It has been normal practice
in The South Manchester Breast Clinic to use a single intramuscular
injection of 100 mg of testosterone propionate to abort severe attacks
of breast pain. No ill-effects have occurred in open studies and this
contrasts with other drugs such as danazol and bromocriptine. Many
women require two or three courses of treatment to obtain relief with
conventional treatment[5]. Women treated in Manchester for premenstrual
tension with subcutaneous implants of testosterone 100 mg noted a
decrease in the severity of their breast pain without significant side-effects

(Anderson, D., personal communication). Testosterone undecanoate (Restandol®, Organon Laboratories Ltd), an oral preparation of testosterone, is rapidly metabolized to the active steroid by first-pass metabolism in the liver. The concentration of testosterone in the serum of women treated with testosterone undecanoate 40 mg b.d. orally is significantly higher than in those treated with placebo (personal communication, Organon Laboratories Ltd). As no placebo-controlled study of testosterone therapy has been reported, it was felt valuable to subject this therapy to a controlled study, which is reported here.

MATERIALS AND METHODS

Following approval by the local ethics committee, 30 women were recruited, using the criteria detailed in Table 1.

After 2 months' preliminary assessment, treatment began on the 1st day of the menstrual period according to a double-blind randomization procedure (Figure 1). The first treatment was given for 12 weeks and patients were then crossed over to the other treatment for a further 12 weeks. The testosterone and identical placebo tablets were supplied by the manufacturer and were dispensed monthly by the local pharmacy.

Table 1 Criteria for admittance to study

(1)	> 21 years old
(2)	Menstrual cycle 21–35 days
(3)	Breast pain > 7 days each cycle not relieved by simple analgesics for at least 3 months
(4)	Pain assessment chart completed for a minimum of 1 month prior to entry
(5)	No biopsy required
(6)	Normal mammogram within 3 months prior to entry for women > 30 years
(7)	Negative pregnancy test prior to treatment
(8)	No planned pregnancy during trial period
(9)	No hormonal preparations within 2 months (i.e. oral contraceptives or danazol)
(10)	No known history of allergy to testosterone undecanoate
(11)	No clinical sign of virilization or hirsutism
(12)	Informed written consent of patient

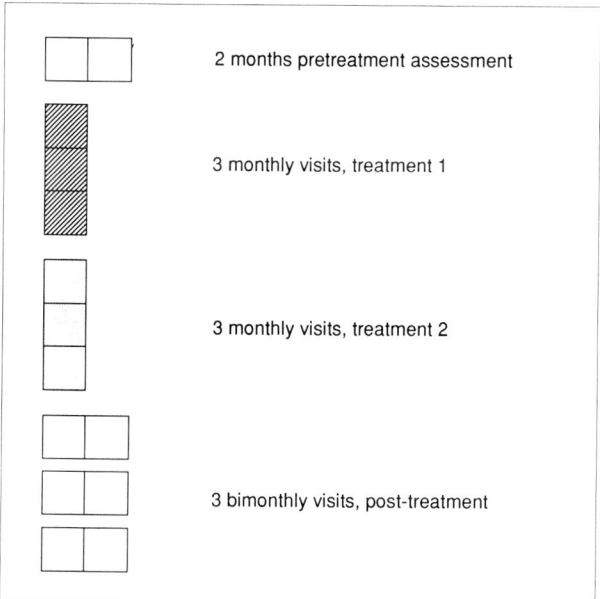

Figure 1   The temporal design of the study

Patients recorded the severity of their pain on visual analogue scales (Figure 2). The patients were assessed clinically at monthly intervals during treatment and for up to three further bimonthly visits after completion of treatment. Pregnancy was excluded when appropriate and adverse effects were monitored. Compliance was checked in two ways: a variable number of tablets were issued each month by the pharmacist and the remaining tablets were counted on each return visit, and radioimmunoassay of serum testosterone was performed. Patients were withdrawn from the trial if any of the following occurred: hypersensitivity to the drug, hypertension, excessive weight gain, metromenorrhagia, virilization or pregnancy.

Analysis

Data were analysed by repeated measures analysis of variance using the GLIM 3.77 computer program. A normal distribution was assumed.

Friday
No pain _____ Worst pain
Period {   }
Other ....

Saturday
No pain _____ Worst pain
Period {   }
Other ....

Sunday
No pain _____ Worst pain
Period {   }
Other ....

Monday
No pain _____ Worst pain
Period {   }
Other ....

Tuesday
No pain _____ Worst pain
Period {   }
Other ....

Wednesday
No pain _____ Worst pain
Period {   }
Other ....

Thursday
No pain _____ Worst pain
Period {   }
Other ....

Is your pain Better {   },   Worse {   }, or the Same {   } as last week?

Figure 2 The weekly proforma used by patients to record their pain, menstrual history and associated symptoms

Order groups were analysed separately. In this preliminary analysis, no account was taken of any cycle effects.

RESULTS

The data show significant changes with time (Table 2). There was a significant reduction ($p \leq 0.001$) of pain scores over each 28-day period in women treated with placebo and testosterone undecanoate. Reduction of pain scores occurred over the worst 7 consecutive days ($p \leq 0.001$) and the best seven consecutive days ($p \leq 0.001$). These reductions occurred irrespective of treatment order. The greatest reduction in pain scores occurred during treatment with testosterone undecanoate.

Three patients were withdrawn; one conceived after 3 months of treatment (on placebo) and two withdrew for persistent nausea. Four patients suffered nausea, the first being the pregnant patient. In a second patient it persisted throughout treatment with placebo and until the 2nd month of treatment with testosterone. A third patient reported nausea whilst taking testosterone and, despite marked reduction in pain, was

Table 2 Reduction in pain scores in women treated with placebo or testosterone undecanoate

	Reduction in pain score	
	Mean	95% confidence limits
Score over total period		
pretreatment	50	37–63
placebo	33	15–42
testosterone undecanoate★	26	9–35
Scores over worst 7 days		
pretreatment	73	53–91
placebo	48	30–67
testosterone undecanoate★	37	21–54
Scores over best 7 days		
pretreatment	50	37–63
placebo	33	15–42
testosterone undecanoate★	26	9–35

★$p \leq 0.001$

withdrawn. A fourth patient experienced mild nausea throughout the trial and the follow-up period but declined withdrawal as she had a favourable response. One patient became amenorrhoeic although follicle stimulating hormone and luteinizing hormone remained within the normal range and menstruation returned 14 months later. Whilst taking testosterone, two patients reported increased libido, one of whom also noted a mild increase in the hair on her upper lip. These effects resolved within 2 months when treatment ceased.

One patient reported abolition of and two patients a marked reduction in premenstrual tension associated with favourable response to testosterone. There were no adverse effects on weight or blood pressure.

DISCUSSION

Few women require therapy for cyclical breast pain, but for those with severe persistent symptoms there are only a limited number of effective treatments and these are frequently associated with adverse effects. Although no allowance has been made for cycle effects, in this preliminary analysis, a clear effect of treatment was demonstrated with a greater decrease in perceived pain while on testosterone undecanoate, irrespective of the order of treatments. Adverse effects occurred to treatment with placebo and testosterone. However, only nausea in two patients and an increased libido and facial hair in a further patient were attributable to testosterone. This low incidence of adverse effects compares favourably with that of other effective hormonal agents used in the treatment of cyclical breast pain[6]. Further evaluation of testosterone undecanoate for the treatment of persistent severe cyclical breast pain is justified.

ACKNOWLEDGEMENTS

We are grateful to Organon Laboratories for support. The secretarial and nursing staff in the Breast Unit at University of South Manchester gave unstinting help.

REFERENCES

1. Haagensen, C.D. (1971). Women's role in recognizing the symptoms of breast disease. In Haagensen, C.D. (ed.) *Diseases of the Breast*, pp. 373–7. (Philadelphia: Saunders)
2. Hinton, C. (1986). Breast pain. In Blamey, R.W. (ed.) *Complications in the Management of Breast Disease*, pp. 231–8. (London: Ballière Tindall)
3. Mansel, R. (1986). Breast pain: clinical spectrum and management. In Forbes, V.F. (ed). *Clinical Surgery International*, Vol. 10, pp. 48–58. (Edinburgh: Churchill Livingstone)
4. Wang, D.Y. and Fentiman, I.S. (1985). Epidemiology and endocrinology of benign breast disease. *Breast Cancer Res. Treatment*, **6**, 5–36
5. Griffith, C.D.M. (1987). The breast pain clinic: a rational approach to classification and treatment of breast pain. *Postgrad. Med. J.*, **63**, 547–9
6. Pye, J.K., Mansel, R.E. and Hughes, L.E. (1985). Clinical experience of drug treatments for mastalgia. *Lancet*, **2**, 373–7

5

Danazol in benign breast disease with clinical, radiographic and thermographic monitoring

*E. Alvarez Gardiol, A. Alvarez Gardiol, J. Alvarado Velloso,
A. Benitez Gil, O. Carbone, R. Venier and U. Questa*

INTRODUCTION

Benign breast disease is a common clinical condition which may present in a variety of ways with varying histopathology. The aetiology remains unknown, although it is usually accepted that it arises as a result of hormonal and environmental factors in conjunction with a genetic predisposition. There is no general agreement on the definition of benign breast disease, nor is there consensus on its role as a true nosological entity. Despite this, the problem is so great that a significant number of women require symptomatic treatment.

The best results are obtained with hormonal treatments and there is a rich bibliography describing the use of danazol. In a non-controlled study, we found that 200 mg danazol per day for 6 months achieved a good symptom response and was fairly well tolerated by patients. In addition, since there is no suggestion that danazol has any influence on breast cancer, we were confident that this treatment would not obscure the diagnosis, in any patient, of an undetected, underlying neoplasia.

SUBJECTS AND METHODS

The female subjects were 60 consenting patients aged between 25 and 45 years who had had symptomatic benign breast disease for 1 year or more. All the patients had diffuse bilateral disease with no clinical or radiological findings indicating the need for breast biopsy.

Excluding criteria for the study were; any features suggestive of breast cancer, any previous history of breast cancer, a breast biopsy within the preceding 5 years, parturition less than 24 months earlier, associated disease in another system, and any hormonal treatment less than 6 months before the start of the study.

Each patient received 100 mg danazol per day for 2 months commencing on the 1st day of the menstrual cycle. After 2 months the patients underwent double-blind randomization to receive placebo (Group I), 100 mg danazol per day (Group II) or 200 mg danazol per day (Group III) for the subsequent 2 months.

Patients underwent interview, clinical examination, mammography and telethermography before the start of the trial and were evaluated thereafter at monthly intervals for the next 7 months, with a final evaluation 360 days after the start of treatment (Table 1). The criteria for grading pain duration and intensity, breast nodule extension and type, mammograms and thermograms are given in Table 2.

Statistical analysis

The Wilcoxon test was used to detect paired differences, and the Friedman test, and the Kruskal–Wallis test for detection of, respectively, differences within, and amongst groups.

RESULTS

The results are given for the 45 women who completed the trial and who were equally distributed amongst the three groups.

Duration and intensity of pain

Figures 1 and 2 show that in all three groups, both the intensity and duration of pain were significantly reduced after 60 days. This improvement continued at 120 days and there was no significant difference between the three groups.

Table 1 Outline of scheme for clinical trial

Days since treatment	Evaluation	Procedure
0	1st interview	full medical history taken, physical examination, mammography, telethermography of breasts performed at a constant ambient temperature $(20 \pm 2°C)$
30	1st evaluation	patient questionnaire, physical examination, ponderal index calculated
60	2nd evaluation	patient questionnaire, physical examination, ponderal index, telethermography
90	3rd evaluation	patient questionnaire, physical examination, ponderal index
120	4th evaluation	patient history of condition, physical examination, mammography, telethermography
150	5th evaluation	patient questionnaire, physical examination, ponderal index
180	6th evaluation	patient questionnaire, physical examination, ponderal index
210	7th evaluation	patient history of condition, physical examination, mammography, telethermography
360	final evaluation	physical examination, mammography and telethermography

The distribution and type of breast nodules

The extension of the breast nodules had been significantly reduced by 60 days in all groups (Figure 3). In Group I after 90 days the distribution of breast nodules did not differ significantly from initial values, whilst throughout the study, the three groups did not differ significantly between themselves.

Table 2 Grading of criteria used to assess outcome

Pain duration
0	no pain
1	pain appears 4 days before menstrual cycle
2	pain appears 5–8 days before menstrual cycle
3	pain appears 9–15 days before menstrual cycle
4	constant pain

Pain intensity
0	no pain
1	aches when touched
2	pain worsened by moving and walking
3	spontaneous pain
4	intolerable pain

Extension of nodules
0	no nodules
1	isolated nodules
2	nodules predominantly in the upper external quadrant
3	nodules predominantly retroareolar
4	multiple nodules throughout breast

Type of breast nodules
0	none
1	cystic
2	solid
3	indeterminate

Mammography
1	minimal radiodensity
2	moderate radiodensity
3	intense radiodensity, condensing opacities

Breast telethermography
1	normal vascular pattern and calibre. No hyperthermic focus
2	normal vascular pattern with increased vascular calibre. Some hyperthermic areas with a temperature gradient of less than 2°C
3	vascular design and calibre or the presence of hyperthermic disorders representing a temperature gradient of more than 2°C

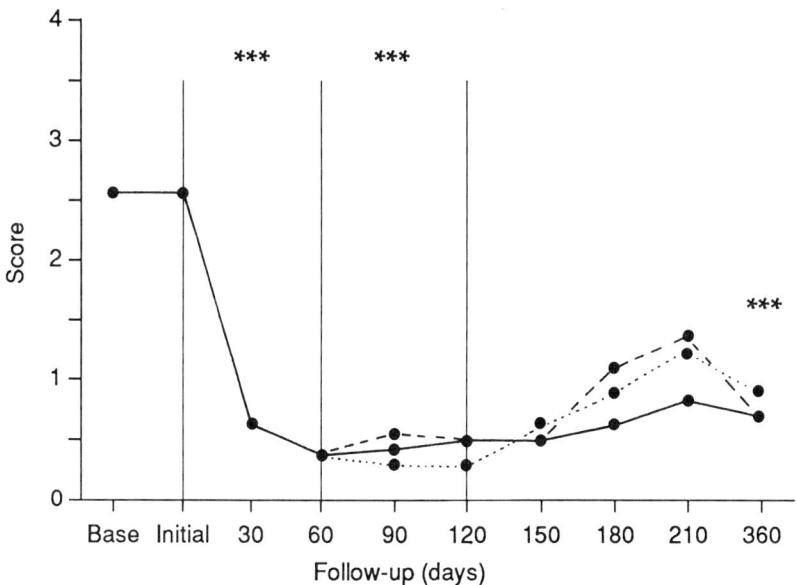

Figure 1 Modifications in the duration of pain. Group I (placebo), ———; Group II (100 mg/day danazol), ————; Group III (200 mg/day danazol), ·····. ***, $p < 0.001$

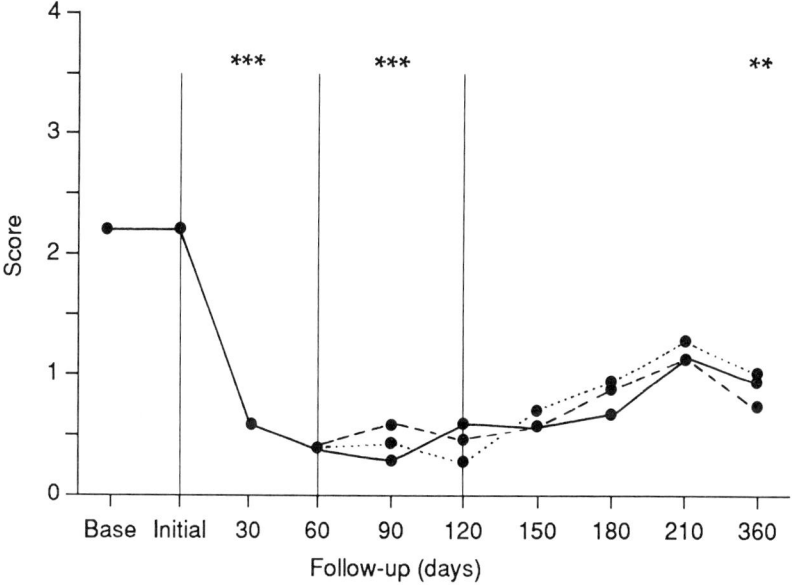

Figure 2 Modifications in the intensity of pain. Group I, ———; Group II, ————; Group III, ·····. **$p < 0.01$; ***, $p < 0.001$

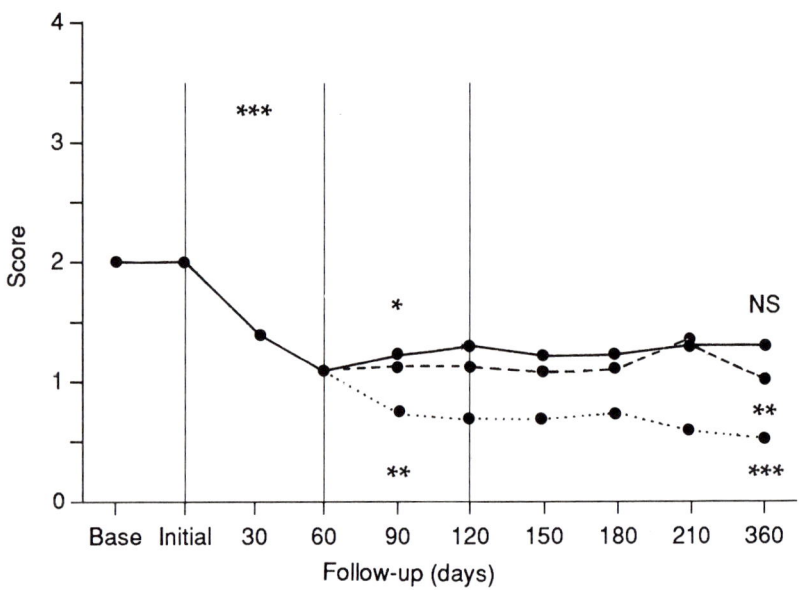

Figure 3 Modifications in the extension of the nodules. Group I, ———; Group II, ————; Group III, ·····. *, $p < 0.1$; **, $p < 0.01$; ***, $p < 0.001$

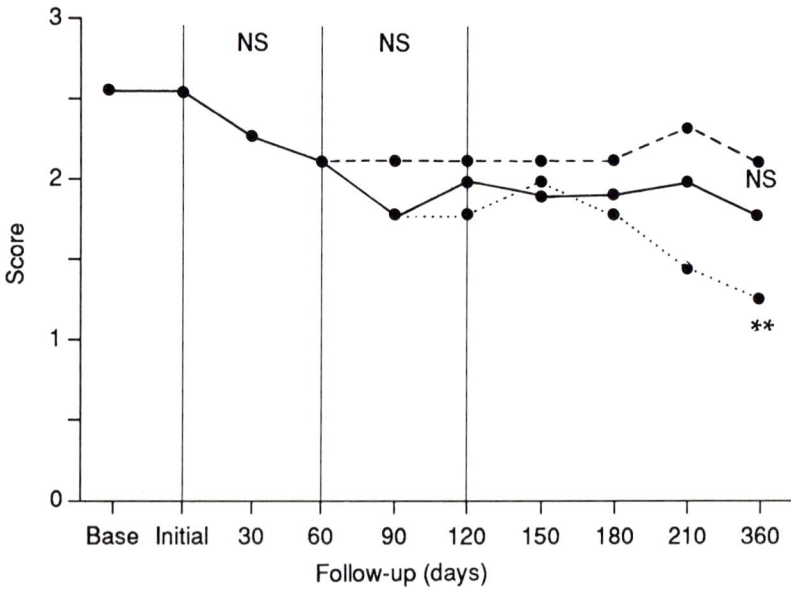

Figure 4 Modifications in the type of the nodules. Group I, ———; Group II, ————; Group III, ·····. **, $p < 0.01$

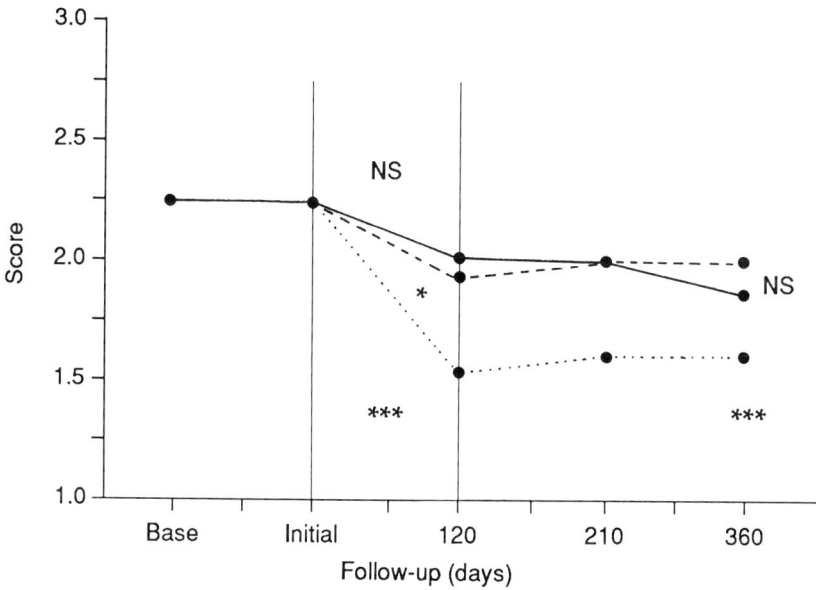

Figure 5 Modifications in the results from mammography. Group I, ———; Group II, ————; Group III, · · · · . *, $p < 0.05$; ***, $p < 0.001$

There was no significant difference in the type of breast nodules (except, surprisingly, in the final evaluations for Group III) in any of the three groups at any point in the study (Figure 4).

Mammography

Group III was the only group to show a significant improvement in the mammographic results and this was seen at 120, 210 and 360 days (Figure 5). Despite this, there were no statistical differences, in the mammographic findings amongst the three groups.

Telethermography

In all three groups, score values at 60, 120, 210 and 360 days differed dramatically from the baseline value. Again there were no significant differences amongst the groups (Figure 6).

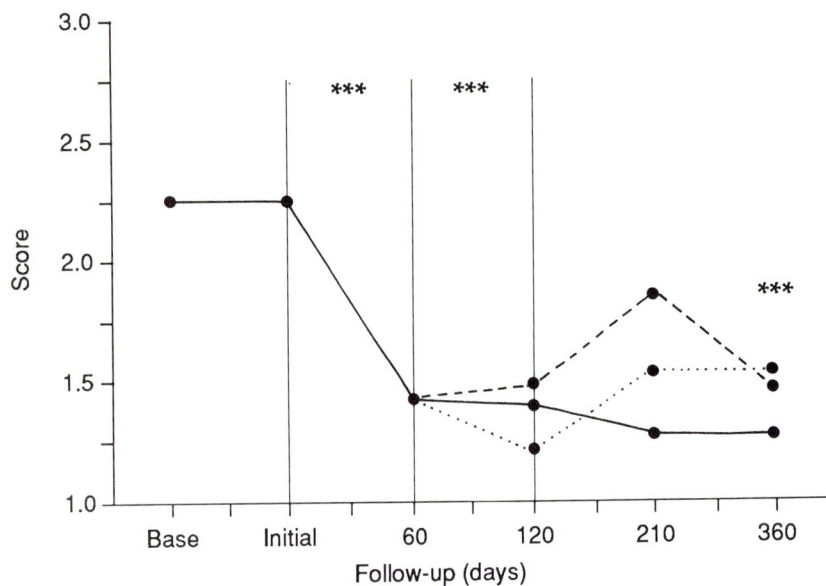

Figure 6   Modifications in vascular calibre by telethermography. Group I, ———;
Group II, ————; Group III, · · · · . ***, $p < 0.001$

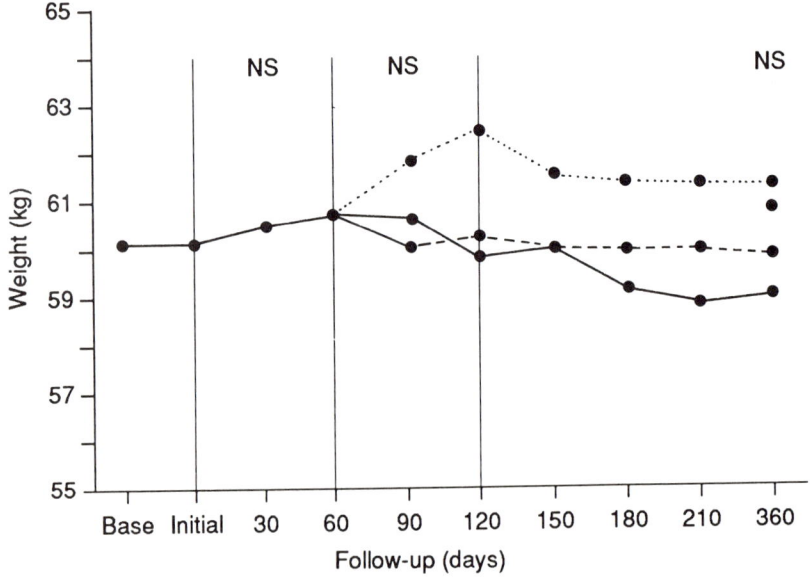

Figure 7   Changes in body weight. Group I, ———; Group II, ————; Group III, · · · ·

Table 3 Side-effects and effects on menstrual cycle seen after treatment with danazol

	Number of patients affected
Side-effect	
None	17
Ankle oedema	8
Diffuse alopecia	3
Headaches	3
Upper limb parasthesia	3
Nausea	1
Spontaneous abortion	1
Pelvic pain	1
Seborrhoea	1
Seasickness	1
Effect on menstrual cycle	
None	28
Early menstruation	10
Polymenorrhoea	4
Scant menstruation	3
Suppression of menstruation	2
Metromenorrhagia	2

ADVERSE EFFECTS OF DANAZOL TREATMENT

Weight gain

Overall, there were no significant differences between initial and final (360 day) body weights in all three groups, or between all three groups, except for Group III which, at the mid-stage of treatment, showed a significant weight gain (Figure 7).

Other side-effects of treatment and effects on menstrual cycle are listed in Table 3.

DISCUSSION

A dose of 100 mg danazol per day for 60 days appears to be very effective at reducing both the intensity and the duration of pain in benign breast disease. Prolonging this treatment, or increasing the dose of danazol does not appear to influence breast symptoms.

Dose and duration of treatment with danazol may be related to a reduction in breast nodules, since patients in group I gradually stopped showing a reduction in nodules after 90 days. The results are even more confused when the type of nodule is considered due to the subjective nature of clinical assessment. Ultrasonography could provide a more accurate assessment in this case.

Changes in breast radiodensity seem to be dependent upon danazol dosage and duration. Even though the three groups did not differ significantly amongst themselves, Group III, with its higher dose, is the one showing the greatest improvements.

Thermographic improvement with danazol at 100 mg/day for 60 days correlated well with improvement in breast symptoms. Consequently, although its use in cancer detection is controversial, thermography could perhaps be used to help follow-up patients with benign breast disease.

CONCLUSION

Danazol at 100 mg per day over 2–4 months is an efficient treatment for benign breast disease. When no clinical response is obtained, both the dose and the duration of treatment should be increased. The treatment appears to be cost effective, with only slight side-effects which are fully reversible on cessation of treatment.

6

The Cardiff Mastalgia Clinic experience of the drug treatments for mastalgia

C.A. Gateley, M. Miers and R.E. Mansel

INTRODUCTION

Breast pain or mastalgia produces a significant medical work load, being the commonest breast complaint seen by general practitioners and accounting for 45–50% of referrals to breast clinics[1]. After exclusion of overt pathology and reassurance the majority of patients need no further treatment. However, in around 15% of those presenting, the severity of pain affects the quality of life and drug treatment should be considered[2]. Placebo-controlled studies of drug treatment in mastalgia have shown a significant response to placebo treatment. Therefore only drugs proven by such studies should be considered for use in mastalgia. Danazol[3,4], bromocriptine[5,6] and evening primrose oil[7] have been tested in such trials and are the drugs used routinely in the Cardiff Mastalgia Clinic.

PATIENTS AND METHODS

Drug treatment is not usually considered until mastalgia has been present for at least 6 months and is of such severity as to affect the quality of life. Assessment of severity is based on subjective reporting of the degree of pain and the effect on the patient's work, sleep and sex life, and objectively by the patients completing a breast pain chart[8]. Completion of the pain chart also allows classification into cyclical and non-cylical mastalgia[9]. If severe pain persists, the therapeutic options are discussed with the patient and the chosen drug started. The patient is reassessed after 2 months' treatment and response graded using the Cardiff Breast Score (CBS) as follows:

(1) CBS I, no pain;

(2) CBS II, substantial response leaving easily bearable pain;

(3) CBS III, poor response leaving substantial pain; and

(4) CBS IV, no response.

CBS I–II are considered to be clinically useful responses. If a clinically useful response has not been obtained after 2 months' treatment with danazol or bromocriptine, or after 4 months' treatment with evening primrose oil, the drug is stopped, the patient reassessed and treatment substituted if appropriate. In this review, if patients did not complete such a therapeutic trial they were not included in the analysis of response to treatment, but were included in the analysis of side-effects.

RESULTS

A total of 414 patients received a therapeutic trial of treatment between 1973 and 1990. Of these 324 had cyclical and 90 non-cyclical mastalgia.

Cyclical mastalgia

As first-line therapy 145 patients were treated with danazol, 94 with bromocriptine and 85 with evening primrose oil. The results of treatment are shown in Table 1.

Treatment of patients who failed to obtain a clinically useful response to first-line drug treatment has been reported previously[10]. Of the patients with cyclical mastalgia, 84 received a second drug treatment after failing on first-line therapy and 48 (57%) obtained a clinically useful response. Of the 20 patients who received a third drug treatment after failing on first- and second-line therapies, five (25%) obtained a

Table 1 First–line response to drug treatment for mastalgia showing numbers of patients in each category

	Danazol	Bromocriptine	Evening primrose oil
Cyclical			
treated	145	94	85
useful response	115 (79%)	51 (54%)	49 (58%)
Non-cyclical			
treated	40	18	32
useful response	16 (40%)	6 (33%)	12 (38%)

clinically useful response. The results of second-line treatment are shown in Table 2[10].

Non-cyclical mastalgia

As first-line therapy 40 patients were treated with danazol, 18 with bromocriptine and 32 with evening primrose oil. The results of treatment are shown in Table 1.

Of the patients with non-cyclical mastalgia, 42 received a second drug treatment after failing on first-line therapy and 10 (24%) obtained a clinically useful response. Out of the 19 patients who received a third drug treatment after failing on first- and second-line therapies, four (21%) obtained a clinically useful response. The results of second-line treatment are shown in Table 3[10].

Table 2 Cyclical mastalgia, useful response to second-line therapy after failure of first-line drug treatment[10]

Second-line treatment	First-line failure		
	Danazol	Bromocriptine	Evening primrose oil
Danazol	—	19/25 (76%)	15/19 (79%)
Bromocriptine	5/15 (33%)	—	4/6 (67%)
Evening primrose oil	1/10 (10%)	4/9 (44%)	—

Table 3 Non-cyclical mastalgia, useful response after failure of first-line drug treatment[10]

| Second-line treatment | First-line failure | | |
	Danazol	Bromocriptine	Evening primrose oil
Danazol	—	3/8 (38%)	3/8 (38%)
Bromocriptine	3/13 (23%)	—	0/3
Evening primrose oil	1/8 (13%)	0/2	—

Adverse events

A total of 752 treatment courses were prescribed (some patients receiving more than one course of treatment). Altogether 295 received danazol, 216 bromocriptine and 241 evening primrose oil. The incidence of significant side-effects is shown in Table 4.

DISCUSSION

This review of the drug treatment of mastalgia from a single centre, using well-defined classifications of pain and response grading, allows comparison of the relative response rates to drug treatment in clinical practice. Cyclical mastalgia is more responsive to treatment than non-cyclical mastalgia, with danazol being the most effective drug for both conditions. Danazol remains equally effective after the failure of bromocriptine and evening primrose oil. Bromocriptine and evening primrose oil may be used after the failure of each other, anticipating the same response rates as if used as first-line therapy. If used after the

Table 4 Significant side-effects in patients receiving drug treatment for mastalgia

	Danazol	Bromocriptine	Evening primrose oil
Patients treated	295	216	241
Side-effects	88 (30%)	75 (35%)	9 (4%)
Treatment stopped because of side-effects	43	46	5

failure of danazol, bromocriptine and evening primrose oil are unlikely to produce a clinically useful response.

These response rates have to be balanced against the side-effects of the three treatments. Significant side-effects are complained of in about one-third of patients treated with danazol and bromocriptine. Danazol may be reduced to a low-dose regimen, after a useful response has been obtained, which decreases the incidence of side-effects[11]. Bromocriptine must be initiated with an incremental build-up, as side-effects are commonly experienced on starting treatment and may resolve if the patient is able to continue with treatment. The incidence of side-effects with evening primrose oil is very small, being no greater than that of placebo treatment in control trials[12].

Therefore, in making the choice of the optimal drug treatment for patients with mastalgia, the chances of obtaining a clinically useful response have to be balanced against the potential side-effects. Effective drug treatments are now available for cyclical and non-cyclical mastalgia, and should be considered in severe cases where the quality of the patient's life is affected.

ACKNOWLEDGEMENT

We thank Mrs E. Lewis who has volunteered her time to the Cardiff Mastalgia Clinic since its inception.

REFERENCES

1. Hughes, L.E., Mansel, R.E. and Webster, D.J.T. (1989). *Benign Disorders and Diseases of the Breast*, pp. 75–92. (London: Baillière Tindall)
2. Pye, J.K., Mansel, R.E. and Hughes, L.E. (1985). Clinical experience of drug treatments for mastalgia. *Lancet*, **2**, 373–6
3. Mansel, R.E., Wisbey, J.R. and Hughes, L.E. (1982). Controlled trial of the antigonadotropin danazol in painful nodular benign breast disease. *Lancet*, **1**, 928–30
4. Hinton, C.P., Bishop, H.M., Holliday, H.W., Doyle, P.J. and Blamey, R.W. (1986). A double blind controlled trial of danazol and bromocriptine in the management of severe cyclical breast pain. *Br. J. Clin. Pract.*, **40**, 326–30
5. Durning, P. and Sellwood, R.A. (1982). Bromocriptine in severe cyclical breast pain. *Br. J. Surg.*, **69**, 248–9

6. Mansel, R.E. and Dogliotti, L. (1990). European multicentre trial of bromocriptine in cyclical mastalgia. *Lancet*, **1**, 190–3

7. Mansel, R.E., Pye, J.K. and Hughes, L.E. (1990). Effects of essential fatty acids on cyclical mastalgia and noncyclical breast disorders. In Horrobin, D. (ed.) *Omega-6 Essential Fatty Acids, Pathophysiology and Roles in Clinical Medicine*, pp. 557–66. (New York: Wiley-Liss)

8. Gateley, C.A. and Mansel, R.E. (1990). Management of cyclical breast pain. *Br. J. Hosp. Med.*, **43**, 330–2

9. Maddox, P.R. and Mansel, R.E. (1989). Management of breast pain and nodularity. *World J. Surg.*, **13**, 699–705

10. Gateley, C.A., Maddox, P.R., Mansel, R.E. and Hughes, L.E. (1990). Mastalgia refractory to drug treatment. *Br. J. Surg.*, **77**, 1110–12

11. Harrison, B.J., Maddox, P.R. and Mansel, R.E. (1989). Maintenance therapy of cyclical mastalgia using low-dose danazol. *J.R. Coll. Surg. Edinb.*, **34**, 79–81

12. Mansel, R.E., Gateley, C.A., Harrison, B.J., Melhuish, J., Sheridan, W., Pye, J.K., Pritchard, G., Maddox, P.R., Webster, D.J.T. and Hughes, L.E. (1990). Effects and tolerability of n-6 essential fatty acid supplementation in patients with recurrent breast cycles. *J. Nutr. Med.*, **1**, 195–200

7

Dietary intervention trials in subjects with benign breast disease

N.F. Boyd, M. Cousins, V. McGuire, G. Lockwood and D. Tritchler

INTRODUCTION

Breast cancer incidence and mortality vary widely around the world and the disease is approximately seven times more common in women in Europe and North America than in women in Japan and other Asian countries[1]. International differences in disease rates are not due to inherited differences between populations, but rather to some environmental difference, because migrants who move from high-risk to low-risk countries acquire the breast cancer incidence of their adoptive country[2]. This change in risk may take two or more generations, as with Japanese migrants to the United States[3] or may take place more quickly, as it has with Polish migrants to the USA and Italian migrants to Australia[4]. Further, breast cancer rates within some low-risk countries have changed substantially over time[1]. For example, increases in age-specific breast cancer incidence have been observed in Japan and Iceland, providing additional evidence that environmental factors can influence breast cancer risk. Although the identity of the environmental factors that influence breast cancer risk is presently unknown there are reasons, discussed below, for believing that diet may be one of them.

DIETARY FAT AND BREAST CANCER RISK

Animal evidence

Animal experiments which show that dietary fat intake influences mammary carcinogenesis have been the subject of several recent reviews[5-7]. Increasing dietary intake of fat is associated with an increase in the number of animals that develop tumours, an increase in the number of tumours that develop per animal and, in experiments involving carcinogens, a reduction in the latent interval before the appearance of tumours. The effects of dietary fat intake on mammary carcinogenesis have been demonstrated in several rodent models involving spontaneous, carcinogen-induced and hormone-induced tumours. The effects of dietary fat on mammary carcinogenesis appear to be greater with unsaturated than with saturated fatty acids. However, some long-chain unsaturated fatty acids, such as eicosapentanoic acid, may inhibit carcinogenesis. Dietary fat appears to act at the promotional stage of carcinogenesis and the demonstrated effects of high fat diets include an increase in the size of transplanted mammary tumours. Some studies have suggested that high fat diets may also have an influence on tumour initiation.

The mechanism of action of high fat diets on mammary carcinogenesis is not well understood. Although an effect of dietary fat on the secretion of some hormones, such as oestrogen and prolactin has been suggested, experimental evidence indicates that such changes cannot explain the effects of dietary fat on the development of mammary tumours. There is some evidence indicating that dietary fat may influence the proliferative activity and responsiveness to mammotropic hormones of mammary epithelial cells[8].

Although animal experiments clearly show that dietary fat intake influences mammary carcinogenesis, it is at present unknown to what extent these data apply to humans. In the following section, the human evidence concerning dietary fat intake and breast cancer risk is considered.

Human evidence

In contrast to animal evidence, human evidence concerning a relationship between dietary fat intake and breast cancer risk is inconsistent. Correlational studies, designs that are generally regarded as being more susceptible to uncontrollable bias or confounding than cohort or case–control studies, have more consistently shown associations between fat intake and breast cancer risk[9]. Strong study designs (cohort and case–control studies) have, however, failed to consistently demonstrate an association between fat consumption and breast cancer risk. Although several investigators have found evidence of an association between fat intake and breast cancer risk, the relationship has usually been weak compared to correlation studies (see references 10–14 for recent reviews).

Epidemiological investigation of the role of fat in breast cancer differs from most other aetiological studies in that there is no group available that has not had some exposure to the agent under study. Investigators are therefore, only able to examine the risk of breast cancer in relation to the extent of exposure, as assessed by the quantity of fat ingested. If, in cohort and case–control studies, populations are examined whose fat intake is systematically less variable than the variation in fat consumption between countries, then the associations found between fat intake and breast cancer risk will be weaker than those found in international correlation studies, if they can be identified at all.

The potential effects of this methodological limitation are illustrated in Figure 1. In this figure, the variability in fat intake which was seen in the most rigorous cohort study reported to date, that of Willett[15], is contrasted with that seen in the only international correlation study which provided data on both fat intake and breast cancer incidence (Gray and colleagues[16]). Breast cancer incidence and per capita fat intake in the 22 countries included in Gray's correlation study were plotted and the least squares regression line fitted to the data. The scale on the abscissa showing percentage calories from fat was fitted by establishing two points, 39% of calories from fat from Willett's data for the USA, and 15% of calories from fat for Japan from the data provided by Kagawa[17]. A linear scale was then constructed between these points.

As shown in Figure 1, the approximately five-fold international variation observed in breast cancer incidence is strongly associated with differences in estimated fat consumption ($r = 0.78$). To estimate the differences in cancer incidence that might be found in association with fat intake within a country, if the international data indeed do indicate a causal association, we have projected onto the regression line the range in fat intake reported in Willett's cohort study. Fat intake varied from 32% of calories (mean of lowest quintile) to 44% of calories (mean of highest quintile). As shown in the figure, this range of fat intake would be expected to be associated with relatively small differences in cancer incidence and the ratio of the risks, in the highest and lowest quintiles as assessed by diet records, would be only 1.4. Misclassification will

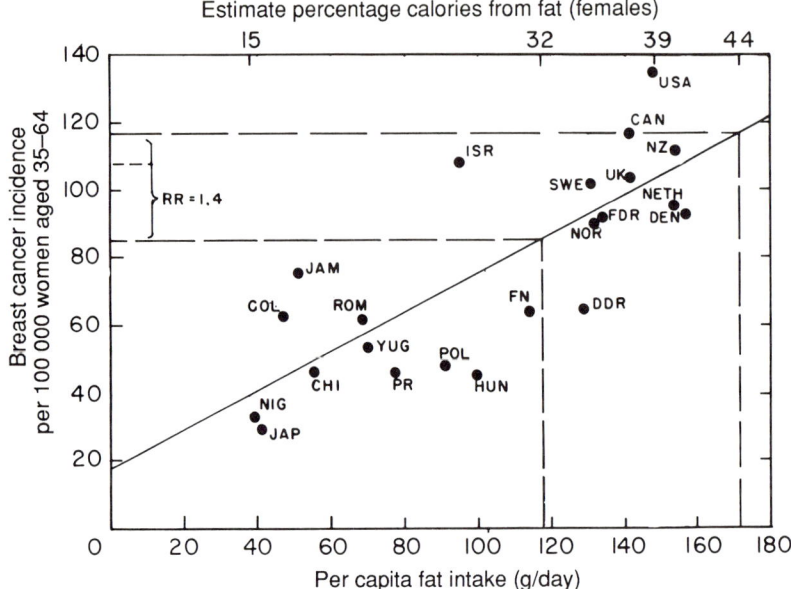

Figure 1 Estimate of the breast cancer risk detectable within the Western population in association with dietary fat. CAN = Canada; CHI = Chile; COL = Columbia; DDR = German Democratic Republic; DEN = Denmark; FDR = Federal Republic of Germany; FN = Finland; HUN = Hungary; ISR = Israel; JAM = Jamaica; JAP = Japan; NETH = The Netherlands; NIG = Nigeria; NOR = Norway; NZ = New Zealand; POL = Poland; PR = Puerto Rico; ROM = Romania; SWE = Sweden; UK = United Kingdom; USA = United States; YUG = Yugoslavia; RR = ratio of risks

reduce the apparent difference in risk between the upper and lower quintiles compared to the 'true' difference in risk, so that the true ratio of 1.4 will appear to be only 1.16[14].

Further study of the relationship between dietary fat and breast cancer risk is required before dietary recommendations can be made concerning this disease. Controlled clinical trials in which the range of fat intake is increased beyond that seen in most Western populations, are capable of overcoming the limitations of observational epidemiology, and would provide the strongest evidence available concerning the relationship of dietary fat intake to breast cancer risk. Further, such trials are the only methods likely to answer the question of whether breast cancer risk in high-risk subjects can be modified by changing dietary fat intake.

Previous work has been concerned with several aspects of the feasibility of an experimental approach to this problem, including the identification of subjects at increased risk for breast cancer, and the demonstration that such subjects will enter a clinical trial of dietary fat reduction and comply with a low fat diet. Preliminary results of an intervention with dietary fat reduction in subjects with mammographic dysplasia have been presented elsewhere[18-20], as has more detailed consideration of the rationale and logistics of this approach[21].

While carrying out this clinical trial, we noted that patients with cyclical mastopathy, a condition that appears to be associated with mammographic dysplasia[22], frequently experienced striking relief of symptoms after reduction of dietary fat. Similar findings have been reported by Rose in an uncontrolled study[23]. We therefore carried out a second trial whose purpose was to test the hypothesis that symptoms of cyclical mastopathy are relieved by a reduction in dietary fat accompanied by an increase in complex carbohydrate[22] that has been reported in detail.

DIETARY FAT REDUCTION AND CYCLICAL BREAST PAIN

A total of 21 patients with severe and persistent cyclical mastopathy were recruited and randomly allocated to a dietary intervention. Subjects were randomly allocated to receive one of two types of dietary advice. A group of controls was given general advice about maintaining a healthy diet according to Canada's Food Guide but were not counselled to change the composition of their diets. The average fat intake of this group was 34% of total calories. A second group was given advice and education about reducing dietary fat intake to 15% of total calories. In both groups the severity of breast tenderness and swelling were assessed monthly using daily diaries, modified from the Cardiff diary.

The principles of the dietary intervention involved the preparation of an individualized dietary prescription, based on a careful assessment of the patient's eating habits at entry to the study, in which fat was substituted by the isocaloric exchange of complex carbohydrate. Patients were encouraged to introduce these dietary principles into their diet as soon as possible, and to adopt the new diet fully within 4 weeks. In addition, we provided several dietary aids that included dietetic scales, a food guide containing the subject's individualized meal pattern, daily food allowance, and additional information such as exchange lists for fat, cereals, fruits and vegetables, an extensive shoppers' guide, suggestions for eating away from home, and approximately 200 low-fat high-carbohydrate recipes.

After randomization, women in the intervention group were seen once every month for 6 months, and those in the control group every 2 months for 6 months. At each visit both groups provided a record of foods eaten on 3 randomly selected days. The principal method of assessing compliance was the nutrient analysis of food records. In addition, serum cholesterol was measured in all patients at randomization and at intervals afterwards corresponding to the collection of food records.

Nutrient changes seen in both groups are shown in Table 1. Total fat intake in the intervention group fell from a mean of 34% of calories at baseline to a mean of approximately 21% of calories after randomization, which was maintained for 6 months. Carbohydrate consumption increased in the intervention group from 47% of calories at baseline to 60% of calories. No changes were observed in the intake of alcohol, caffeine or α-tocopherol (data not shown).

Changes in the severity of breast swelling and tenderness during the course of the study are shown in Figure 2. Results are expressed as the difference in severity scores recorded in the diaries for the postmenstrual (day 7) and premenstrual (2 days before the onset of menstruation) phases of the cycle, the absence of a difference indicating an absence of cyclical changes in these symptoms.

As Figure 2 shows, there was, in the intervention group, a striking reduction in the severity of cyclical breast swelling and tenderness over the course of 6 months. Statistical assessment by analysis of variance of these changes in the 18 patients for whom complete data were available gave p values of 0.0399 ($F(3,14) = 3.63$) for breast swelling and 0.0001 ($F(3,14) = 18.37$) for breast tenderness. These changes in self-reported symptom severity were similar to those found by a physician who interviewed these subjects.

Details of the biochemical changes noted in this trial have been given elsewhere[24]. Plasma levels of oestrone, oestradiol and progesterone were similar in both groups throughout the study. Levels of sex hormone

Table 1   Mean intake of selected nutrients; % means percentage of total calories

Nutrient	Baseline	2 months	4 months	6 months
Energy (kcal)				
study	1693	1474	1352	1491
control	1690	1857	1744	1676
Protein (%)				
study	14.9	16.1	16.6	17.9
control	16.2	18.2	7.0	15.8
Total fat (%)				
study	33.6	21.4	20.1	22.8
control	36.2	37.0	37.2	33.4
Saturated fat (S) (%)				
study	13.0	7.4	7.2	8.8
control	13.5	14.1	15.3	12.3
Polyunsaturated fat (P) (%)				
study	6.3	4.7	4.1	4.0
control	7.5	6.8	6.2	7.4
P/S ratio				
study	0.57	0.82	0.71	0.61
control	0.62	0.56	0.44	0.66
Total carbohydrate (%)				
study	47.1	59.1	56.9	56.3
control	45.3	41.1	44.1	48.1
Alcohol (%)				
study	6.1	5.5	8.7	4.8
control	3.9	5.1	3.0	4.2
Caffeine (%)				
study	318	340	284	285
control	268	258	246	249

binding globulin and prolactin did not differ significantly between the groups at any time.

Serum cholesterol did not differ significantly between the groups at any time but statistically significant changes within the intervention did occur that were close to those predicted. Changes in consumption of

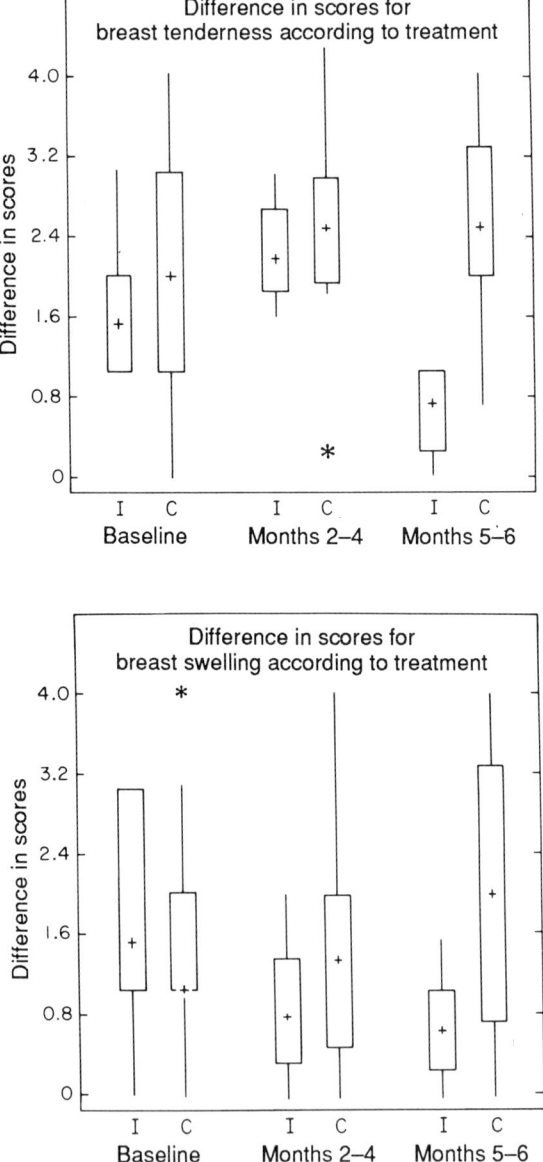

Figure 2 Box plots showing differences in the severity of premenstrual and postmenstrual breast tenderness (upper figure) and breast swelling (lower figure) in intervention and control groups at baseline, 3 and 6 months after randomization

total energy ($r = 0.76$, $p = 0.02$), total fat ($r = 0.69$, $p = 0.04$), saturated fat ($r = 0.65$, $p = 0.06$), polyunsaturated fat ($r = 0.68$, $p = 0.04$), protein ($r = 0.90$, $p = 0.0009$) and dietary cholesterol ($r = 0.75$, $p = 0.02$) were all significantly correlated with change in the severity of the symptom of breast tenderness at 6 months.

None of the hormonal measurements (oestrone, oestradiol, progesterone, prolactin or sex hormone binding globulin) showed evidence of an association with change in symptoms but change in serum cholesterol did show an association that was of borderline statistical significance ($r = 0.69$, $p = 0.06$).

PLASMA LIPIDS AS POSSIBLE MARKERS OF BREAST CANCER RISK

The possibility that plasma lipids might be associated with distinctive breast cancer risk was raised during earlier work in which we measured plasma lipids and lipoproteins in women with mammographic dysplasia, who were taking part in the clinical trial of dietary fat reduction referred to above. Comparison of the values obtained with age- and sex-specific values for the population showed that values for total cholesterol did not differ notably from those expected. Values for high density lipoprotein cholesterol (HDL-C) were, however, skewed markedly towards the upper end of the distribution for the population, and 50% of the values fell at or above the 75th percentile for women of the same age. Triglycerides and low density lipoprotein cholesterol (LDL-C) both showed a distribution that was skewed towards the lower end of the distribution expected in the population.

To examine this finding further, we compared premenopausal women with different patterns of the breast parenchyma on mammography. One group had extensive radiological dysplasia ($n = 30$) and the other no dysplasia ($n = 16$). Both groups were recruited from mammographic units in the same way and then compared according to epidemiological risk factors, anthropometric measures, nutrient intake, and plasma levels of oestradiol, progesterone and prolactin obtained in both follicular and luteal phases of the menstrual cycle, as well as total plasma cholesterol and lipid fractions.

Women with mammographic dysplasia were found to be leaner, more often nulliparous, and to consume more alcohol than women without these radiological changes. Mammographic dysplasia and a family history of breast cancer were found to be independently associated with significantly higher levels of HDL-C after taking into account the possible confounding effects of body fat percentage, parity and consumption of alcohol and dietary fat. Triglyceride levels were also independently associated with a family history of breast cancer. No differences were found in plasma levels of oestradiol, progesterone, or prolactin[25].

Plasma levels of HDL-C were highest in subjects with both mammographic dysplasia and a family history of breast cancer, lowest in those with neither of these attributes and intermediate in women with mammographic dysplasia but no family history. Triglyceride levels were also influenced by both of these variables, but in the opposite direction.

These findings suggest that the mammographic densities referred to as dysplasia are associated with an alteration in lipid metabolism. It is of interest, therefore, that several treatments for benign breast disease also influence plasma lipids. In particular, danazol, which has been shown to reverse the radiological appearance of dysplasia[26], has been reported to lower plasma levels of HDL-C by about 40%[27-29].

Examination of the relationship of HDL-C to other epidemiological features of breast cancer shows several additional points of similarity. Adult women in Western society have higher plasma levels of HDL-C than men and this difference is influenced by female sex hormones[30]. Puberty in females is associated with higher levels of plasma HDL-C than in males[31]. Measurements of HDL-C levels in different countries show that in general HDL-C levels are higher in women in countries where the risk of breast cancer is also high[32-34].

Parity is known to reduce breast cancer risk and a recent large cohort study conducted in Belgium showed that HDL-C levels are lower in parous than nulliparous women and that HDL-C levels are approximately 40% lower after pregnancy than before[35].

Several studies, including the one described above, have shown that a reduced fat diet reduces HDL-C and raises triglyceride levels in healthy premenopausal women[36-40]. Observational surveys show that HDL-C level is associated with dietary practices, and suggest that differences in diet are responsible for the difference in HDL-C levels found between countries that were referred to above[41,42].

Alcohol consumption has been found consistently to increase risk of breast cancer[43] and there is an abundant literature showing that alcohol consumption raises HDL-C levels[44]. Body weight appears to exert different effects on breast cancer risk before and after the menopause. Risk of premenopausal breast cancer is associated with normal or lean body type[45], whereas postmenopausal risk appears to be increased by obesity[46]. HDL-C has been found to be negatively correlated with body weight both before and after the menopause[47].

A recent large cohort study from the Lipid Research Clinics showed that risk of death from 'gynaecologic cancer' (most due to breast cancer) changed approximately 23% for every 10 mg/dl difference in baseline HDL-C level[48].

It is clearly not possible in the present state of knowledge to state whether HDL-C or apoprotein AI are more likely to be markers of breast cancer risk or to play some direct role in causing the disease. However, in serum free culture systems HDL-C and apoprotein AI have been shown to control cell proliferation, an activity that may be relevant to carcinogenesis[49,50].

CONCLUSIONS AND SUGGESTIONS FOR FUTURE WORK

An intervention involving a substantial reduction in dietary fat intake with an increase in complex carbohydrate results in striking symptom relief in women with severe cyclical breast tenderness and swelling. The influence of a low-fat high-carbohydrate diet on symptoms of cyclical mastopathy suggests that fat has short-term physiological effects on the breast. These effects should be more precisely characterized, in view of the evidence that dietary fat and premenstrual breast symptoms may be related to breast cancer risk[51-53]. The development of physical methods of characterizing breast tissue would obviously help considerably in elucidating these effects and magnetic resonance imaging is now being assessed from this point of view.

The biochemical changes found to be associated with mammographic dysplasia and other risk factors for breast cancer suggest that plasma lipids, particularly HDL-C, may be a marker of breast cancer risk, and plasma levels of HDL-C are influenced by a number of other risk factors for breast cancer, including dietary fat.

Interest in the relationship of HDL-C to disease has so far been concerned primarily with its protective role in coronary heart disease. The results shown here, as well as data in the literature, suggest that further investigation is warranted regarding the role of HDL-C in relation to breast cancer risk. The association of plasma lipid levels with other risk factors for breast cancer should be examined, including studies of the association with familial risk for the disease and the association of lipid levels with histological changes that confer increased risk. A large-scale dietary intervention study in women with mammographic dysplasia would allow examination of the effect of a dietary change which lowers HDL-C levels on breast cancer risk. Although HDL-C levels and coronary heart disease risk are negatively correlated within countries, they are positively correlated between countries[54]. Dietary fat reduction would therefore be expected to lower heart disease risk even though HDL-C levels are reduced. For example, the 'Prudent diet' currently recommended by the American Heart Association has been shown to lower HDL-C levels[55].

REFERENCES

1. Doll, R. and Peto, R. (1981). *The Causes of Cancer: Quantitative Estimates of Avoidable Risks of Cancer in the United States.* (Oxford: Oxford University Press)
2. Buell, P. (1974). Changing incidence of breast cancer in Japanese-American women. *J. Natl. Cancer Inst.*, **51**, 1479–83
3. Kmet, J. (1970). The role of migrant populations in studies of selected cancers. *J. Chron. Dis.*, **23**, 305–24
4. Haenzel, W. (1970). Studies of migrant populations. *J. Chron. Dis.*, **23**, 289–31
5. Welsch, C.W. (1986). Interrelationship between dietary fat and endocrine processes in mammary gland tumorigenesis. *Prog. Clin. Biol. Res.*, **222**, 623–54
6. Rogers, A.E. and Lee, S.Y. (1986). Chemically induced mammary gland tumors in rats: modulation by dietary fat. *Prog. Clin. Biol. Res.*, **222**, 255–82

7. Freedman, L.S., Clifford, C. and Messina, M. (1990). Analysis of dietary fat, calories, and body weight and the development of mammary tumours. *Cancer Res.*, **50**, 5710–19

8. Welsch, C.W., DeHoog, J.V., O'Conner, D.H. and Sheffield, L.G. (1985). Influence of dietary fat levels on development and hormone responsiveness of the mouse mammary gland. *Cancer Res.*, **45**, 6147–54

9. Prentice, R., Kakar, F., Hursting, S., Sheppard, L., Klein, R. and Kushi, L.H. (1988). Aspects of the rationale for the Women's Health Trial. *J. Natl. Cancer Inst.*, **80**, 802–14

10. Willett, W.C. (1989). The search for the causes of breast and colon cancer. *Nature (London)*, **338**, 389–94

11. Schatzkin, A., Greenwald, P., Byar, D.P. and Clifford, C. (1989). The dietary fat–breast cancer hypothesis is alive. *J. Am. Med. Assoc.*, **261**, 3284–7

12. Cohen, L.A. (1987). Diet and cancer. *Sci. Am.*, **257**, 42–8

13. Rose, D.P. (1986). Dietary factors and breast cancer. *Cancer Surv.*, **3**, 671–87

14. Goodwin, P. and Boyd, N.F. (1987). A critical appraisal of the evidence that dietary fat intake is related to breast cancer risk in humans. *J. Natl. Cancer. Inst.*, **79**, 473–85

15. Willett, W.C., Stampfer, M.J., Colditz, G.A., Rosner, B.A., Hennekens, G.H. and Speizer, F.E. (1987). Dietary fat and the risk of breast cancer. *N. Engl. J. Med.*, **316**, 22–8

16. Gray, G.E., Pike, M.C. and Henderson, B.E. (1979). Breast-cancer incidence and mortality rates in different countries in relation to known risk factors and dietary practices. *Br. J. Cancer*, **39**, 1–7

17. Kagawa, Y. (1978). Impact of Westernization on the nutrition of Japanese: changes in physique, cancer, longevity and centenarians. *Preventive Med.*, **7**, 205–17

18. Boyd, N.F., Cousins, M., Beaton, M., Fishell, E., Wright, B., Fish, E., Kriukov, V., Lockwood, G., Tritchler, D., Hanna, W. and Page, D. L. (1988). Clinical trial of low fat, high carbohydrate diet in subjects with mammographic dysplasia: report of early outcomes. *J. Natl. Cancer Inst.*, **80**, 1244–8

19. Lee-Han, H., Cousins, M., Beaton, M., McGuire, V., Kriukov, V., Chipman, M. and Boyd, N. (1988). Compliance in a randomized clinical trial of dietary fat reduction in patients with breast dysplasia. *Am. J. Clin. Nutr.*, **48**, 575–86

20. Boyd, N.F., Cousins, M., Beaton, M., Kuriov, V., Lockwood, G. and Tritchler, D. (1988). Relationship between dietary change and serum cholesterol in women: results from a randomized controlled trial. *Am. J.*

Clin. Nutr., **52**, 470–6

21. Boyd, N.F., Cousins, M., Lockwood, G. and Tritchler, D. (1990). The feasibility of testing experimentally the dietary fat–breast cancer hypothesis. *Br. J. Cancer*, **62**, 878–81

22. Leinster, S.J., Whitehouse, G.H. and Walsh, P.V. (1987). Cyclical mastalgia: clinical and mammographic observations in a screened population. *Br. J. Surg.*, **74**, 220–2

23. Rose, D.P., Boyar, A., Haley, N., Cohen, L.A., Lahti, H. and Strong, L.E. (1985). Low fat diet in fibrocystic disease of the breast with cyclical mastalgia: a feasibility study. *Am. J. Clin. Nutr.*, **42**, 856

24. Boyd, N.F., McGuire, V., Shannon, P., Cousins, M., Kriukov, V., Mahoney, L., Fish, E., Lickley, L., Lockwood, G. and Tritchler, D. (1988). The effect of a high fat low carbohydrate diet on symptoms of cyclical mastopathy. *Lancet*, **2**, 128–32

25. Boyd, N.F., McGuire, V., Fishell, E., Kriukov, V., Lockwood, G. and Tritchler, D. (1989). Plasma lipids in premenopausal women with mammographic dysplasia. *Br. J. Cancer*, **59**, 766–71

26. Asch, R.M. and Greenblatt, R.B. (1977). The use of an impeded androgen – danazol – in the management of benign breast disorders. *Am. J. Obstet. Gynecol.*, **127**, 130–4

27. Luciano, A.A., Hauser, K.S. and Sherman, B.M. (1983). Effects of danazol on plasma lipid and lipoprotein levels in normal women. *Atherosclerosis*, **43**, 133–7

28. Schewepe, K.W. and Assmann, G. (1984). Changes of plasma lipids and lipoprotein levels during danazol treatment for endometriosis. *Horm. Metab. Res.*, **16**, 593–7

29. Fahraeus, L., Larsson-Cohn, U., Ljungberg, S. and Wallentin, L. (1984). Profound alterations of lipoprotein metabolism during danazol treatment for endometriosis. *Fertil. Steril.*, **42**, 52–7

30. Lipid Research Clinics Program Epidemiology Committee (1979). Plasma lipid distribution in selected North American populations. *Circulation*, **60**, 427–39

31. Srinivasan, S.R., Sundaram, G.S., Williamson, G.D., Webber, L.S. and Berenson, G.S. (1985). Serum lipoproteins and endogenous sex hormones in early life: observations in children with different lipoprotein profiles. *Metabolism*, **34(9)**, 861–7

32. Kesteloot, H., Huang, D.X., Yang, X.S., Claes, J., Rosseneu, M., Geboers, J. and Joossens, J.V. (1985). Serum lipids in the People's Republic of China: comparison of Western and Eastern populations. *Arteriosclerosis*, **5**, 427–33

33. Halfon, S.T., Rifkind, B.M., Harlap, S., Kaufmann, N.A., Baras, M.,

Slater, P.E., Halperin, G., Eisenberg, S., Davies, A.M. and Stein, Y. (1980). Plasma lipids and lipoproteins in adult Jews of different origins: The Jerusalem Lipid Research Clinic Prevalence Study. *Isr. J. Med. Sci.*, **18**, 1113–20

34. Punnonen, R., Jokela, H., Kudo, R., Punnonen, K., Pyykko, K. and Pystynen, P. (1987). Serum lipids in Finnish and Japanese postmenopausal women. *Atherosclerosis*, **68**, 241–7

35. van Stiphout, W.A.H., Hofman, A. and de Bruijn, A.M. (1987). Serum lipids in young women before, during and after pregnancy. *Am. J. Epidemiol.*, **126**, 922–8

36. Jones, D.Y., Judd, J.T., Taylor, P.R., Campbell, W.S. and Nair, P.P. (1987). Influence of caloric contribution and saturation of dietary fat on plasma lipids in premenopausal women. *Am. J. Clin. Nutr.*, **45**, 1451–6

37. Kuusi, T., Ehnholm, C., Huttunen, J.K., Kostainen, E., Pietinen, P., Leino, U., Uusitalo, U., Nikkari, T., Iacono, J.M. and Puska, P. (1985). Concentration and composition of serum lipoproteins during a low fat diet at two levels of polyunsaturated fat. *J. Lipid Res.*, **26**, 360–7

38. Brussaard, J.H., Dallinga-Thie, G., Groot, P.H.E. and Katan, M.B. (1980). Effects of amount and type of dietary fat on serum lipids, lipoproteins and apoproteins in man. *Atherosclerosis*, **36**, 515

39. Ehnholm, C., Huttenen, J.K., Pietinen, P., Leino, U., Mutanen, M., Kostainen, E., Pikkarainen, J., Dougherty, R., Iacono, J. and Puska, P. (1982). Effect of diet on serum lipoproteins in a population with a high risk of coronary heart disease. *N. Engl. J. Med.*, **307**, 850–5

40. Shepherd, J., Packard, C.J., Patsch, J.F., Gotto, A.M. and Taunton, O.D. (1978). Effects of dietary polyunsaturated and saturated fat on the properties of high density lipoproteins and the metabolism of apoprotein AI. *J. Clin. Invest.*, 1582

41. Sacks, F.M., Castelli, W.P., Donner, A. and Kass, E.H. (1975). Plasma lipids and lipoproteins in vegetarians and controls. *N. Engl. J. Med.*, **292**, 1148–51

42. Tamir, D., Edelstein, P., Reshef, A., Halfon, S. and Palti, H. (1987). Serum cholesterol (total, low density lipoprotein cholesterol, and high density lipoprotein cholesterol) triglyceride levels and fat consumption among Jerusalem Arab and Jewish schoolchildren. *Preventive Med.*, **16**, 752–60

43. Graham, S. (1987). Alcohol and breast cancer risk. Editorial, *N. Engl. J. Med.*, **316**, 1211–12

44. Williams, P.T., Krauss, R.M., Wood, P.D., Albers, J.J., Dreon, D. and Ellsworth, N. (1985). Association of diet and alcohol intake with high density lipoprotein subclasses. *Metabolism*, **34**, 524–30

45. Willet, W.C., Browne, M.L., Bain, C. *et al.* (1985). Relative weight and

risk of breast cancer among premenopausal women. *Am. J. Epidemiol.*, **122**, 731–40

46. de Waard, F., Cornelius, J.P., Aoki, K. and Yoshida, M. (1977). Breast cancer incidence according to weight and height in two cities of the Netherlands and in Aichi prefecture, Japan. *Cancer*, **40**, 1269–75

47. Heiss, G., Johnson, N.J., Reiland, S. *et al.* (1980). The epidemiology of plasma high density lipoprotein cholesterol levels. The Lipid Research Clinics Program Prevalence Study. *Circulation*, **62** (Suppl. IV), 116–36

48. Cowan, L.D., O'Connell, D.L., Criqui, M.H. *et al.* (1990). Cancer mortality and lipid and lipoprotein levels: the lipid research clinics program mortality follow-up study. *Am. J. Epidemiol.*, **131**, 468

49. Gospodarowicz, D., Lui, G.-M. and Gonzalez, R. (1984). High density lipoproteins and the proliferation of human tumour cells maintained on extracellular matrix-coated dishes and exposed to defined medium. *Cancer Res.*, **42**, 3704–13

50. Jozan, S., Faye, J.C., Tourmier, J.F. *et al.* (1985). Interaction of estradiol and high density lipoproteins on proliferation of the human breast cancer cell line MCF-7 adapted to grow in serum free conditions. *Biochem. Biophys. Res. Commun.*, **133**, 105–12

51. Wynder, E.L., MacCornack, F.A. and Stellman, S.D. (1978). The epidemiology of breast cancer in 785 United States caucasian women. *Cancer*, **41**, 2341–4

52. Kaplan, S.D. and Acheson, R.M. (1966). A single etiologic hypothesis for breast cancer? *J. Chron. Dis.*, **19**, 1221–30

53. Schwartz, D., Denoix, P.F. and Rouguette, C. (1987). Enquete sur l'etiologic des cancers genitaux de la femme. 1. Cancer du sein. *Bull. Assoc. Francais Etude Cancer*, **45**, 476–93

54. Miller, N.E. (1987). Lipoprotein metabolism: a major risk factor for coronary atherosclerosis. *Baillières Clin. Endocrinol. Metab.*, **1**, 603–22

55. Kohlmeier, M., Striker, G. and Schlierf, G. (1988). Influences of 'normal' and 'prudent' diets on biliary and serum lipids in healthy women. *Am. J. Clin. Nutr.*, **42**, 1201–5

8

Non-cyclical breast pain: 1-year audit of an improved classification

M.H. Galea and R.W. Blamey

INTRODUCTION

Mastalgia is the commonest breast symptom presenting to general practitioners[1], but until comparatively recently was one that failed to attract much medical attention or research interest. It was against a background of confusing terminology and ignorance of the aetiology that a mastalgia clinic was established in Cardiff 17 years ago. Since then workers at the Cardiff Mastalgia Clinic have done much to improve our understanding of the classification, natural history and treatment options[2-4]. Above all, what has become clearly apparent is the need to classify patients with mastalgia into homogeneous subgroups so that response to therapies can be assessed[5].

Cyclical breast pain, thought to be an exaggeration of normal premenstrual breast pain and tenderness and of hormonal origin, is relatively straightforward to identify and responds well to endocrine manipulation[6].

The same is not true for non-cyclical breast pain; it is often unilateral, response to endocrine manipulation is poor and classification of women into homogeneous groups has proved more difficult. However, there is now emerging a consensus view that non-cyclical breast pain should be classified principally into 'true' non-cyclical breast pain, and pain of musculoskeletal origin[5]. This differentiation should allow an improved understanding of the aetiology and afford more effective treatment.

With the aim of improving the response to treatment, the classification of non-cyclical breast pain in the Nottingham mastalgia clinic has continued to evolve. This paper describes a classification of non-cyclical breast pain, and the results of treatment using this classification, in women seen in the clinic over the last year.

PATIENTS AND METHODS

In the Nottingham breast referral clinic, approximately 1000 new women with mastalgia are seen per annum. The great majority (> 85%) are reassured after examination and discharged back to the care of their general practitioner. Only those women with symptoms bad enough to interfere with their daily activities, social relationships or sleep are referred on to the mastaglia clinic.

CLASSIFICATION

After questioning and examination, the women are divided into those with cyclical breast pain and those with non-cyclical breast pain. Cyclical breast pain describes breast pain, usually bilateral but often more severe on one or other side, that predominantly occurs premenstrually and is improved by the onset of a period. Non-cyclical breast pain has no such relationship with the menstrual cycle; it may be continuous or intermittent, depending on the underlying aetiology, but the pain is complained of by the woman as coming from the breast.

Non-cyclical breast pain is then further subdivided into five classifications.

Medial chest wall pain

This is invariably localized over the costo-chondral region and equates with the condition labelled 'Tietze's disease'.

Lateral chest wall pain

This condition appears to split equally between localized and diffuse pain. Its distribution is most commonly along the lateral border of the pectoralis major, the anterior–mid axillary line and in apposition to the axillary tail. To establish the diagnosis of lateral chest wall pain, it is often helpful to roll the patient into the lateral position so that the breast falls away from the chest wall.

Cervical spondylosis

This diagnosis refers to a group of women whose breast pain is seen as part of a more generalized pain, with a distribution over the axilla, shoulder, medial arm and sometimes the neck. X-ray of the cervical spine is performed: some radiological abnormality has to be present for this label to be applied.

Duct ectasia

This is a label that describes the complaint of burning or stabbing pains, centred around or under the nipple–areolar complex; there may or may not be other visible signs of duct ectasia and they tend to run an indolent and intermittent course.

Breast trigger spot

On examination women in this subgroup have either a single or occasionally two very localized tender spots within the breast parenchyma. Pain, often stabbing or 'toothache-like', is elicited with gentle palpation.

TREATMENT

Women with localized pain, chest wall or breast trigger spot were offered injection of 1 ml local anaesthetic with 1 ml (40 mg) methylprednisolone acetate into the site of maximal tenderness. These women were reviewed at 1 month.

Patients with diffuse lateral chest wall pain were offered a nonsteroidal anti-inflammatory drug (NSAID), usually naproxen 250 mg t.d.s., for a 6-week period and were reviewed at 2 months. Women with cervical spondylosis were managed with a combination of referral for physiotherapy and NSAID and reviewed at 2 months. The women with duct ectasia were managed with reassurance and analgesia as required, and reviewed at 1 month.

Response to initial treatment was considered beneficial if at review the pain had resolved or markedly improved to the extent that no further treatment was necessary.

RESULTS

Between October 1989 and October 1990, 141 new referrals were seen in the mastalgia clinic. A total of 78, median age 38 years (range 20–52) were considered to have cyclical breast pain. The remaining 63 women were considered to have non-cyclical breast pain. Their median age was 53 years (range 18 80) and 60 of the 63 women had pain that was unilateral. The number of women within each diagnostic classification and the results of treatment using this classification are illustrated in Table 1.

There were no serious side-effects from medication, although some women were not able to tolerate the initial choice of NSAID. Most women with localized pain treated with injection described worsening of their symptoms for 24–72 hours before noticing any improvement.

Table 1 Non-cyclical breast pain: classification and response to treatment. Injection consisted of 1 ml local anaesthetic + 1 ml methylprednisolone acetate

Classification	Therapy	Number of patients	Beneficial response n	%
Medial chest wall pain (localized)	injection	20	14	70
Lateral chest wall pain				
localized	injection	11	7	64
diffuse	NSAID	13	7	53
Cervical spondylosis	physiotherapy with/without NSAID	13	10	77
Duct ectasia	analgesia	4	4	
Breast trigger spot	injection	2	2	

DISCUSSION

It is of no surprise that women with non-cyclical breast pain have a median age higher than women experiencing cyclical breast pain and that the pain is principally unilateral: this has been noted previously[5]. It is surprising however, to find that troublesome non-cyclical breast pain accounted for just under 50% of new referrals over a 1-year period; clearly it is a significant problem especially in the older woman. More importantly it is not well described that 90% of women with this unilateral non-cyclical breast pain do in fact have musculoskeletal pain. Why if pain of musculoskeletal origin is such a common cause of non-cyclical breast pain has it not been widely recognized before?

It is unlikely that the distribution of troublesome mastalgia in the female population in Nottingham is different from elsewhere in the country. Much more probable is that in the mastalgia clinic, having recognized this diagnostic group, we actively search out these women by careful questioning and appropriate examination. The clinician should be alerted to the likely diagnosis after questioning; that the pain may be of musculosketal origin is often suggested by a 'normal breast' examination despite the women's complaining of severe 'breast' pain.

Having labelled 90% of troublesome non-cyclical breast pain as musculoskeletal in origin, what about the underlying aetiology? Cervical spondylosis is due to either disc protrusion in the younger woman or degenerative changes in the older woman. The aetiology of the other chest wall pains, however, remains speculative. Anecdotally, our experience in Nottingham is that many of these women work in jobs that require repetitive daily use of the arm such as seamstresses or domestics, and that there is another group who have associated generalized musculoskeletal aches and pains. In the former group the pain is often diffuse, with marked tenderness over the lateral border of the pectoralis major suggesting a pectoral 'fasciitis'. The localized chest wall pain, if medial, is often referred to as a 'costo-chondritis' although there is no reported histological evidence to back this up; we would advocate describing the pain rather than applying a pathological diagnosis.

Localized chest wall pain was treated with injection of local anaesthetic and methylprednisolone acetate it is likely that other steroid preparations, such as hydrocortisone would be equally effective. Likewise, the decision to use naproxen as the initial NSAID was an empirical one, based on an efficacy vs. side-effects 'best guess'. A number of women did experience side-effects of NSAID and required an alternative choice of NSAID; no women required admission to hospital because of these side-effects.

The classification described has allowed subdivision of women with non-cyclical breast pain into homogeneous groups. This has allowed treatment to be more precise and response to initial treatment to be improved; overall a beneficial response to initial treatment was seen in approximately 70% of women. This compares favourably to initial response rates obtained in women with cyclical breast pain treated with hormone manipulation. It is anticipated that overall response will improve as women failing initial treatment are changed to other therapies.

REFERENCES

1. Roberts, M.M., Elton, R.A., Robinson, S.E. and French, K. (1987). Consultation for breast disease in general practice and referral patterns. *Br. J. Surg.*, **74**, 1020–2

2. Preece, P.E., Hughes, L.E., Mansel, R.E. *et al.* (1976). Clinical syndromes of mastalgia. *Lancet*, **2**, 170–3

3. Wisbey, J.R., Kumar, S., Mansel, R.E. *et al.* (1983). Natural history of breast pain. *Lancet*, **2**, 672–4

4. Pye, J.K., Mansel, R.E. and Hughes, L.E. (1985). Clinical experience of drug treatment for mastalgia. *Lancet*, **2**, 373–7

5. Maddox, P.R., Harrison, B.J., Mansel, R.E. and Hughes, L.E. (1989). Non-cyclical mastalgia: an improved classification and treatment. *Br. J. Surg.*, **76**, 901–4

6. Goodwin, P.J., Neelam, M. and Boyd, N.F. (1988). Cyclical mastopathy: a critical review of therapy. *Br. J. Surg.*, **75**, 837–44

9

Effect of goserelin on bone metabolism in patients with mastalgia

H. Hamed, I. Fogelman, W. Gregory and I.S. Fentiman

INTRODUCTION

Goserelin is a long-acting luteinizing hormone releasing hormone (LHRH) agonist which causes reversible suppression of ovarian hormones to castrate levels. It was initially introduced in the mastalgia clinic at Guy's to treat women with severe breast pain who had failed to respond to other effective agents, and subsequently to treat women with previously untreated and recurrent severe mastalgia. Its efficacy and side-effects are discussed in Chapter 2. It is well established that oestrogen deficiency is a major cause of accelerated bone loss[1]. Therefore a study was conducted to assess the bone metabolism in fundamentally healthy premenopausal women who received goserelin implants for mastalgia.

PATIENTS AND METHODS

A total of 40 otherwise healthy premenopausal women with severe mastalgia who required treatment, and 23 matched controls for age, height, weight and menstrual status were entered into the study. Eligibility criteria and the schedule of treatment are discussed elsewhere[2]. Serial measurements of serum calcium, alkaline phosphatase, osteocalcin and fasting urine calcium/creatinine ratio, together with direct measurements of bone mineral density of femoral neck and lumbar spine (L1–4) using dual energy X-ray absorptiometry were undertaken. Baseline values were used as a reference point for subsequent assessment, and the Wilcoxon paired *t*-test was used to measure the statistical significance.

RESULTS

Both patients and controls were similar in terms of age, weight, and height, as shown in Table 1. Baseline biochemical values and bone mineral density measurements did not differ significantly. Suppression of ovarian hormones was achieved in all treated women and serum oestradiol levels reduced to < 17 pg/ml. One patient had an oestradiol level of 26 pg/ml. All previously menstruating women developed amenorrhoea. A total of 29 patients and 16 controls who had complete data at the end of the treatment period, together with 17 patients and 11 controls with 6 months' follow-up, and eight patients and four controls with 12 months' follow-up were assessed. There were no significant changes in any of the parameters in the control group during the study period. However, among those who received goserelin, there was a statistically significant reduction in bone mass, both in the femoral neck and lumbar spine, at 3% and 5%, respectively at the end of the 6 months' treatment (Figures 1 and 2) (Table 2).

This was associated with a statistically significant increase in serum calcium (Figure 3), calcium/creatinine ratio, serum osteocalcin (Figure 4), and alkaline phosphatase, with maximum values at the end of the 6 months' treatment period. However, none of the patients had serum calcium levels above the upper limit of the normal range. Following

Table 1 Characteristics of patients and controls, given as mean value ± standard deviation

	Patients (n = 40)	Controls (n = 23)
Age (years)	37.3	37.8
Height (cm)	158.7 ± 8.1	160.0 ± 5.4
Weight (kg)	64.4 ± 11.5	59.3 ± 9.8

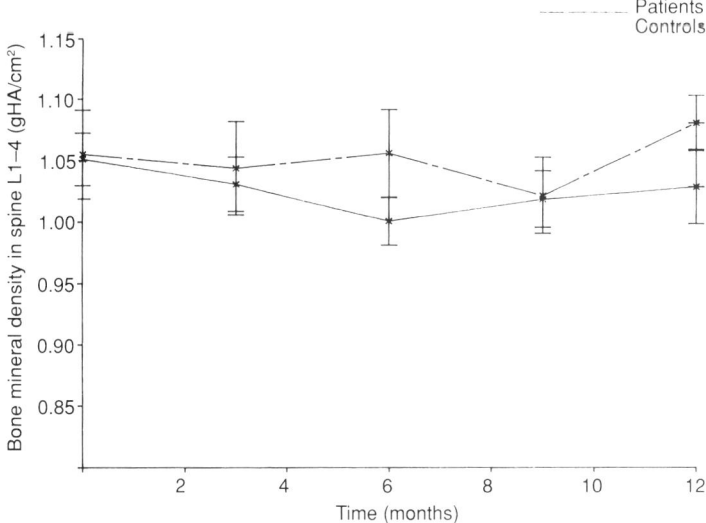

Figure 1 Bone mineral density of lumbar spine, measured over 12 months, in patients taking goserelin and in controls

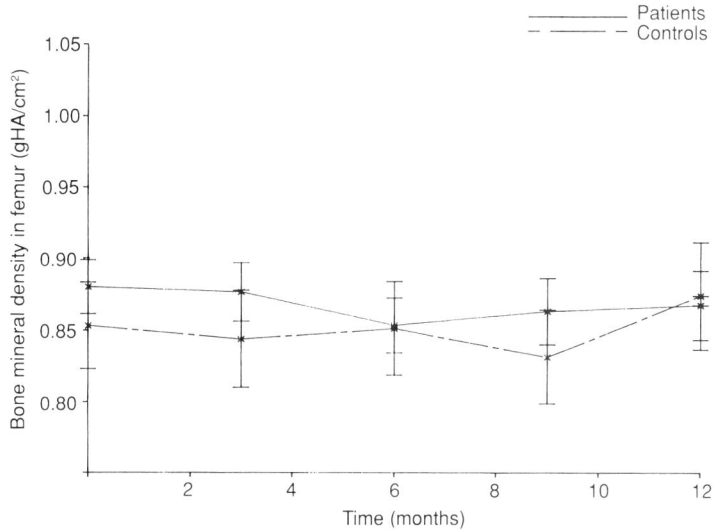

Figure 2 Bone mineral density of femoral neck in patients taking goserelin and in controls

Table 2 Goserelin study: magnitude and significance of differences at 6 and 12 months; + indicates a gain, − indicates a loss

	0–6 months		0–12 months		6–12 months	
	p	Median	p	Median	p	Median
Bone mass						
spine	< 0.001	−0.05 (5%)	0.007	−0.02 (2%)	0.001	+0.03
femur	0.001	−0.02 (3%)	0.02	−0.03 (3%)	0.75	0
Serum calcium	< 0.001	+0.09	0.91	0	0.01	−0.14
Serum alkaline phosphatase	< 0.001	+42	0.002	+13	0.02	−20
Serum osteocalcin	< 0.001	+1	0.008	+0.8	0.35	−0.25
Serum calcium/creatinine ratio	0.08	+0.19	0.05	−0.19	0.02	−0.13

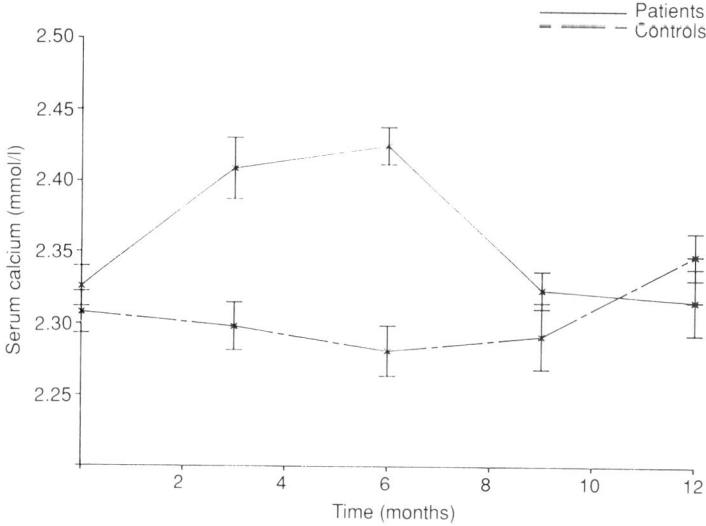

Figure 3   Serum calcium over 12 months in patients taking goserelin and in controls

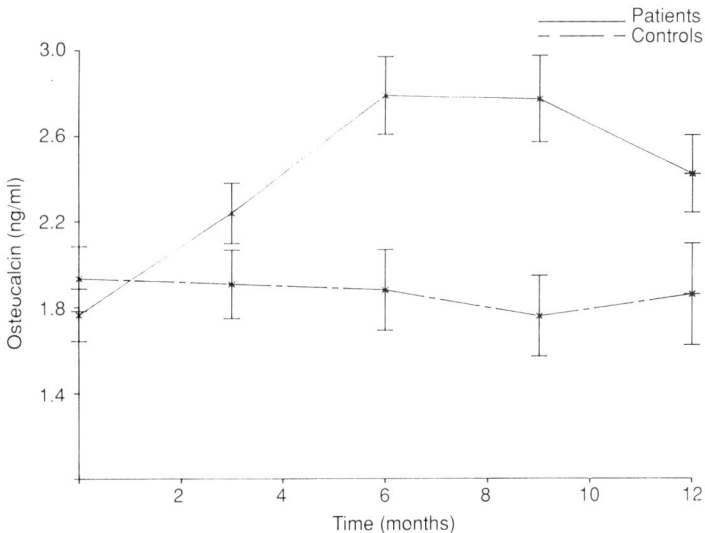

Figure 4   Serum osteocalcin in patients taking goserelin and in controls

cessation of treatment, there was no evidence of further bone loss and indeed there was a slow recovery in both the femoral neck and lumbar spine. However, the values had not returned to baseline levels by the end of the 6 months' follow-up, nor had it recovered in the eight patients who were followed-up for 12 months.

Serum calcium and urine calcium/creatinine ratio declined to baseline levels after 3 months' follow-up. In contrast, serum alkaline phosphatase and osteocalcin remained above the baseline values at 6 months, although levels were lower than those measured at the end of the treatment period (Table 2).

DISCUSSION

These results suggest that chemical castration of females causes bone loss of a similar magnitude to oophorectomy[3]. It was reassuring to observe no further bone loss after stopping treatment, both in terms of direct measurement of bone mineral density, and the return of serum calcium levels and calcium/creatinine ratio to baseline values within 3 months. Serum alkaline phosphatase and osteocalcin have a different significance, being markers of bone turnover, resorption coupled with formation. The decline in the levels of these parameters at the end of the treatment period indicates a slower rate of turnover compared to that during the administration of goserelin. However, sustained high levels suggest that the balance between formation and resorption was not achieved, although formation predominates. In contrast to what has been reported by other investigators, the bone mass in our patients had not completely recovered even after 12 months of cessation of treatment[4]. One explanation could be the marked suppression of oestradiol levels achieved by goserelin implants, in contrast to those achieved by intranasal formulations of LHRH agonists used in other studies[5]. These findings have significant clinical implications, particularly for patients with mastalgia, a characteristically chronic disorder, which may require repeated drug administration. The prolonged phase of bone recovery should be given serious consideration regarding the timing of possible repeated treatment. Goserelin should not be used as first-line treatment for mastalgia since other less toxic therapies are available. Its use should be restricted to patients who have not responded to other forms of treatment.

REFERENCES

1. Lindsay, R., Hart, D.M., Aitken, J.M., MacDonald, E.B., Anderson, J.B. and Clarke, A.C. (1976). Long term prevention of postmenopausal osteoporosis by oestrogen. *Lancet*, **1**, 1038
2. Hamed, H., Caleffi, M., Chaudary, M.A. and Fentiman, I.S. (1990). LHRH analogue for treatment of recurrent and refractory mastalgia. *Ann. R. Coll. Surg. Engl.*, **72**, 221–4
3. Cann, C.E., Genant, K.K., Ettinger, B. and Gordan, G.S. (1980). Spinal mineral loss in oophorectomised women: determination by quantitative computed tomography. *J. Am. Med. Assoc.*, **244**, 2056
4. Waibel-Treber, S., Minne, H.W., Scharla, S.H., Bremen, Th., Ziegler, R. and Leyendecker, G. (1989). Reversible bone loss in women treated with GnRH-agonist for endometriosis and uterine leiomyoma. *Hum. Reprod.*, **4**, 384–8
5. Matta, W.H. and Shaw, R.W. (1987). Hypogonadism induced by luteinising hormone releasing hormone agonist analogue: effects of bone density in premenopausal women. *Br. Med. J.*, **294**, 1523

10

A randomized controlled trial of evening primrose oil for mastalgia

I.D. Campbell, J.C.M. Stewart, G.T. Royle and I. Taylor

INTRODUCTION

Mastalgia is a common problem. It is the commonest reason for a general practice consultation with a breast symptom[1]. It affects some 66% of working women[2], and 50% of patients to a specialist breast clinic[3]. Mastalgia is of sufficient severity to require drug treatment in 8% of such clinic referrals[4].

There is evidence to suggest that mastalgia may be linked to a partial deficiency of essential fatty acids, in particular, the immediate precursors of the prostaglandin E1 series of prostanoids[5,6]. Evening primrose oil (EPO), a vegetable oil produced from selected varieties of evening primrose plants, is a natural source of one of these precursors, γ-linolenic acid (γ-LA). Dietary supplementation with EPO is an attractive form of therapy for mastalgia because it is safe and rarely associated with any adverse effects. The alternative treatments currently available, including danazol, bromocriptine, tamoxifen and goserelin, are commonly associated with significant adverse effects[7]. Three randomized double-blind placebo-controlled studies of EPO have been carried out[8]. All three utilized a visual analogue scale to assess breast pain, completed once each month in the premenstrual period. All showed improvement with EPO compared to pretreatment levels and the placebo groups. When the three trial results were combined, statistical significance was achieved ($2p < 0.0014$, and $2p = 0.011$, respectively). One of the studies showed no further improvement beyond the first 3 months on EPO[9]. Two of the studies suggested that improvement on EPO compared to placebo continued beyond 2 and 5 months, respectively.

The aims of this study are, firstly, to demonstrate whether EPO is significantly better than placebo for cyclical and non-cyclical mastalgia, when treatment is continued for 6 months duration; and, secondly, to assess a different method of symptom assessment, the daily graphic rating scale. The trial is ongoing and this paper presents the methods used and some very preliminary results.

METHODS

Trial design

This study is a parallel randomized double-blind placebo-controlled trial, with a 2-month pretreatment phase for all trial entrants to assess their baseline pattern and severity of symptoms. This is followed by a 6-month treatment phase on either EPO or placebo with 2-monthly clinical assessments.

Medication

Both groups receive eight 500 mg capsules daily in a divided dose according to patient choice. Four capsules twice daily is recommended. The active capsules contain 500 mg EPO (fatty acid content: 9% γ-LA, 73% linoleic acid) plus 10 mg of vitamin E as an antioxidant. Placebo capsules appear identical but contain liquid paraffin. Liquid paraffin is not absorbed and does not noticeably affect bowel function at this dose.

Study population

Trial entrants are derived from women presenting to the Southampton symptomatic breast clinic with breast pain. Women over 18 years of age with at least 6 months' moderate to severe mastalgia, of a cyclical or non-cyclical nature, are referred for trial consideration. Severity is based on patient opinion plus significant interference with daily activities such as sleep, work or movement and physical contact. Malignancy is ruled out by consultant clinical assessment, X-ray- and/or sono-mammography, with aspiration cytology or breast biopsy if indicated.

Women with musculoskeletal pain, those who are pregnant or trying to conceive, postmenopausal or posthysterectomy women, patients suffering from severe intercurrent illness, and those who are epileptic or on phenothiazines or corticosteroids are excluded. Oral contraceptive use is not discontinued but entrants are requested not to change pill during the trial.

Those appropriate for trial inclusion are invited to participate and informed consent is obtained.

Symptom assessment

Graphic rating scales (Figure 1) are used to score symptoms. Breast pain, tenderness, lumpiness, overall symptoms and their relationship to the menstrual cycle are all documented daily by trial entrants. A comments section is included for notes of any adverse effects, new medication and any other symptoms associated with mastalgia, such as breast heaviness or swelling or irritability, which are a particular additional feature of the overall score. Scores are recorded using a vertical mark at any position along the scale and measured in millimetres from the beginning of the scale.

Pain, tenderness and lumpiness are scored by a single investigator (IDC) on identical scales at the 2-monthly clinical assessments. These visits are timed to take place in the last 10 days of the menstrual cycle where possible. Pain scores are based predominantly on patient history, tenderness and lumpiness scores on clinical examination.

An early morning luteal phase blood sample for fatty acid and prolactin levels is taken immediately prior to the start of treatment and following at least 5 months on capsules. Plasma and red cell membrane fatty acid levels are assessed by gas liquid chromatography (GLC) and prolactin levels by conventional radioimmunoassay and by a new bioactive assay (performed in Cardiff).

RESULTS

On the basis of previous work, it was estimated that 40 women would be required to complete the trial, to have a 90% probability of showing a significant effect from EPO.

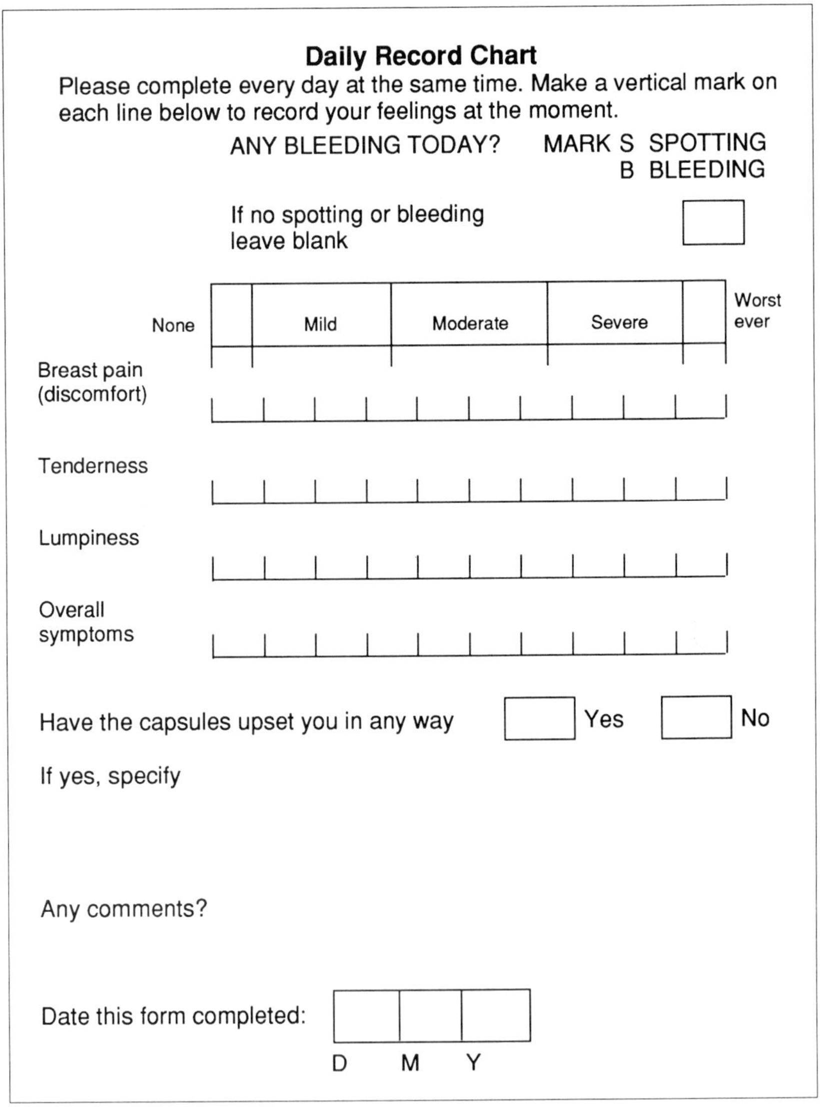

Daily Record Chart

Please complete every day at the same time. Make a vertical mark on each line below to record your feelings at the moment.

ANY BLEEDING TODAY?   MARK S SPOTTING
                                                 B BLEEDING

If no spotting or bleeding
leave blank

| None | | Mild | Moderate | Severe | | Worst ever |

Breast pain
(discomfort)

Tenderness

Lumpiness

Overall
symptoms

Have the capsules upset you in any way   [ ] Yes   [ ] No

If yes, specify

Any comments?

Date this form completed: [| |]
                                              D   M   Y

Figure 1 A page from the daily diary books, demonstrating the graphic rating scales used for symptom assessment

Participation

To date, 163 women have been referred for trial consideration. Of these, 108 women met the inclusion criteria and were prepared to participate in an 8-month randomized trial with its attendant inconveniences. These women commenced the pretreatment phase in which symptoms only were assessed. Three women refused the trial because their breast pain was so bad they wished for immediate definite treatment. Of the 108, 49 women entered the treatment phase of the trial. The major reasons for not entering the treatment phase were:

(1) Pain no longer of sufficient severity after reassurance and negative mammography;

(2) Unknown because of failure to attend follow-up;

(3) Preference to go directly on to EPO, especially since late 1990 when EPO became available on prescription and no longer cost about £25 per 250 capsules.

A total of 44 women have had cyclical mastalgia and five women non-cyclical mastalgia. Ten women in the cyclical group have dropped out of the trial, three because of side-effects, namely headache, nausea on swallowing the capsules and worse breast pain. All three were taking placebo. Two women have become pregnant, one took a travelling job which made attendance for assessment too difficult and four women failed to attend (three on EPO, one on placebo).

Symptom assessment

Participants found the graphic rating scales to be a practical method of symptom assessment and rapidly introduced this and capsule consumption into their daily routines.

The daily graphic rating scale permits analysis of results in several ways: mean scores for the premenstrual phase of the cycle; mean scores over the period of peak symptoms during the cycle, and total area under the curve produced by plotting symptom scores against day of the cycle (Figure 2).

So far, 26 women in the cyclical group have completed the trial and a further two of the women who dropped out were sufficiently far into the treatment phase to permit analysis of results. These numbers are insufficient as yet for publication of differences between the placebo and active groups, except to say that there has been an improvement in both

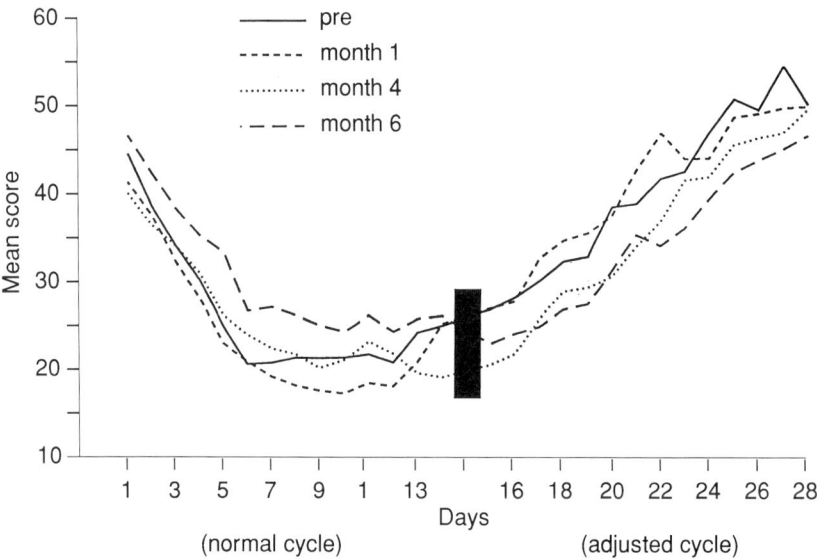

Figure 2 Mean breast pain scores for the 26 women who have completed the trial and for the two withdrawals with adequate information for inclusion, in the pretreatment phase and months 1, 4 and 6 on treatment, using an adjusted menstrual cycle to allow for variation in different women's cycle length. Days 1–14 represent the actual days 1–14. Days 15–28 represent the last 14 days of each woman's cycle. The shaded box represents the region where scores are missing for women with a cycle length of over 28 days

groups for pain and tenderness scores on treatment, with a marked placebo response.

The patterns for pain and tenderness scores in the cyclical group are virtually identical and demonstrate very well the fluctuation of symptoms with the menstrual cycle (Figure 2). Of particular importance, using this method of symptom assessment, is that it can be seen that cyclical mastalgia is not purely a premenstrual condition. Many women experience symptoms during the first 2–3 days of menstruation and indeed the period of worst symptoms frequently extends into this time period.

DISCUSSION

The trial again demonstrates that many women[2,7], after reassurance that their mastalgia symptoms are not due to cancer, are able to cope with their symptoms without further treatment and indeed in some cases the symptoms disappear.

The graphic rating scale has not previously been used for assessment of mastalgia symptoms. It is a modification of the visual analogue scale with the same major advantage, that is, the provision of a sensitive and continuous scale for symptom assessment[10]. In addition the graphic rating scale utilizes the descriptive terms, in this case 'mild', 'moderate' or 'severe'. These may help to reduce the tendency with visual analogue scales of clustering scores on certain parts of the scale[11] and provide a guide to assist consistency of scoring over a long trial period such as this one of 8 months' duration.

Daily assessment has been found to be practical and demonstrates that, although women with cyclical mastalgia have a marked cyclical pattern to their symptoms, in many cases severe and even worst symptoms extend into the first 2–3 days of menstruation. Many previous mastalgia treatment trials have not taken this phase of the cycle into consideration.

The three previous randomized trials of evening primrose oil have used peak premenstrual symptoms to assess results. Work by Kersey and colleagues[12] showed that prospective symptom assessment at one point in the premenstrual period correlated well with their method of prospective daily assessment at this phase of the cycle. The advantage of daily assessment of scores is that analysis is possible of the duration of symptoms as well as amplitude. The duration of symptoms may vary from a few days of the cycle to three or more weeks of the cycle in different women. The full results of this study will be published when 40 women have completed treatment.

REFERENCES

1. Roberts, M.M., Elton, R.A., Robinson, S.E. and French, K. (1987). Consultations for breast disease in general practice and hospital referral patterns. *Br. J. Surg.*, **74**, 1020–2
2. Hughes, L.E., Mansel, R.E. and Webster, D.J.T. (1989). *Benign Disorders and Diseases of the Breast. Concepts and Clinical Management*, pp. 75–92. (London: Baillière Tindall)
3. Smallwood, J.A., Kye, D.A. and Taylor, I. (1986). Mastalgia: is this commonly associated with operable breast cancer? *Ann. R. Coll. Surg.*, **68**, 262

4. Pye, J.K., Mansel, R.E. and Hughes, L.E. (1985). Clinical experience of the drug treatments for mastalgia. *Lancet*, **2**, 373–7

5. Brush, M.G., Watson, S.J., Horrobin, D.F. and Manku, M.S. (1984). Abnormal essential fatty acid levels in plasma of women with premenstrual syndrome. *Am. J. Obstet. Gynecol.*, **150**, 363–6

6. Horrobin, D.F. and Manku, M.S. (1989). Premenstrual syndrome and premenstrual breast pain (cyclical mastalgia): disorders of essential fatty acid (EFA) metabolism. *Prostaglandins, Leukotrienes and Essential Fatty Acids*, **37**, 255–61

7. Preece, P.E. (1990). Mastalgia. In Smallwood J.A. and Taylor, I. (eds.) *Benign Breast Disease*, pp. 44–58. (London: Edward Arnold)

8. Mansel, R.E., Wilkins, D.C. and Preece, P. (1991). Treatment of breast pain by evening primrose oil (Efamast), in press

9. Preece, P.E., Hanslip, J.I., Gilbert, L., Walker, D., Pashby, N.L., Mansel, R.E., Evans, B. and Hughes, L.E. (1982). Evening primrose oil (Efamol) for mastalgia. In Horrobin, D.F. (ed.) *Clinical Uses of Essential Fatty Acids*. (New York: Eden Press)

10. Maxwell, C. (1978). Sensitivity and accuracy of the visual analogue scale: a psychophysical classroom experiment. *Br. J. Clin. Pharmacol.*, **6**, 15–24

11. Dixon, J.S. and Bird, H.A. (1981). Reproducibility along a 10 cm vertical visual analogue scale. *Ann. Rheum. Dis.*, **40**, 87–9

12. Kersey, P., Kruikov, V., Shannon, P. and Boyd, N.F. (1989). Cyclical mastopathy: an evaluation of methods of assessment. *J. Clin. Epidemiol.*, **42**(1), 53–9

11

Symptoms on follow-up of benign breast disease

M.E. Miers and R.E. Mansel

INTRODUCTION

In 1990, 3924 South Wales women were sent a postal questionnaire concerning breast symptoms as part of an ongoing study of breast clinic attenders. The study is a prospective study of the significance of Wolfe mammographic patterns[1] in predicting the risk of future development of a breast cancer. The criteria for entry to the Wolfe study were a mammogram as a result of a breast clinic appointment during the years 1980–85. Two groups of women are being prospectively followed. Those with a breast cancer diagnosis are being followed through clinic attendance to determine the incidence of cancer in the contralateral breast. The method of follow-up for those known not to have had breast cancer is an annual review form which asks study women to report on breast symptoms experienced during the past 12 months, on breast operations, and on mammography.

QUESTIONNAIRE RESULTS

To date, 2802 (71.4%) of 3924 women have returned a breast review form in 1990. There is no significant difference in the response rates for the 6 years of entry, 1980–85. A total of 480 (17.1% of responders) reported a breast symptom during the previous year. These 480 women reported 554 symptoms.

Type of symptom

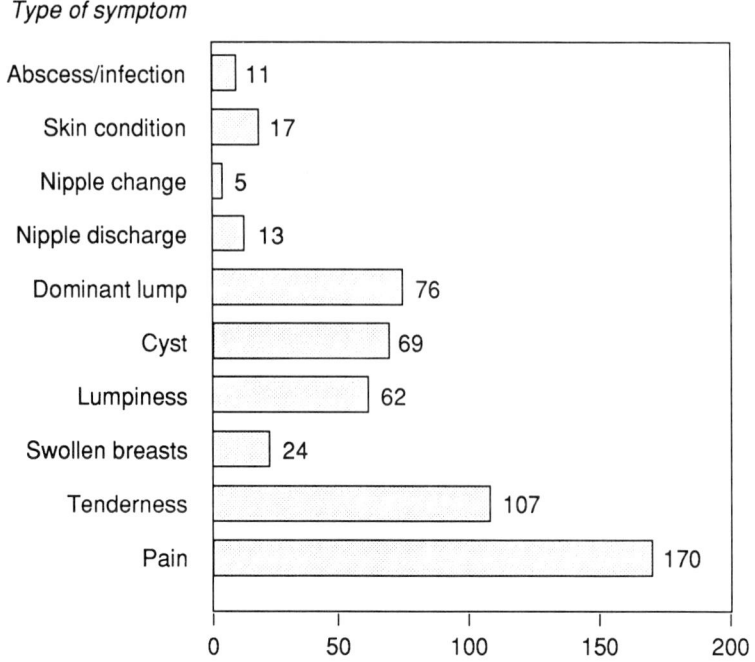

Figure 1 Breakdown of 554 breast symptoms reported by 480 women

Breast pain, the most common complaint, was reported by 170 women (30.3% of the symptoms). Pain, tenderness and swelling together comprised 54.3% of reported symptoms. Of those reporting breast pain, 59 (34.7%) reported that it was related to their menstrual cycle, or to a hormonal change (for example, commencing hormone replacement therapy), and 68 (40%) reported unilateral pain. Pain in the left breast was three times more common than in the right.

A total of 69 women (14.3% of women reporting symptoms) reported cysts (or 'lumps' which were 'drained' or 'aspirated'), and 76 (15.8%) reported discrete lumps. Nipple changes or nipple discharges were noted only 18 times (Figure 1).

Of the discrete lumps, 24 (31.2%) were excised; four were found to be malignant and 12 were histologically normal (see Table 1). Twelve other operations were reported: for mammographic abnormalities (3), for cosmesis (5), for mastalgia (2), for duct ectasia (1), and for reported pain in breast and arm found to be caused by malignancy.

Table 1 Findings in 24 lumps excised in the previous year

'Normal'	12
Cancer	4
Duct ectasia	2
Fibroadenoma	2
Hamartoma	1
Lipoma	1
Sclerosing adenosis	1
Abscess	1

CLINICAL MANAGEMENT

The patients' symptoms were grouped to determine priority for clinical management. Patients who reported symptoms of discrete lumps, nipple changes and nipple discharge were given priority in ensuring further assessment. These patients' hospital records were checked to ensure that they had been clinically assessed. Any women who did not appear to have been seen by a doctor were contacted by letter or telephone. Of the 76 women reporting discrete lumps, 62 (82%) were seen in an outpatient clinic, and 45 (59.2%) required further clinical review. Five women consulted their general practitioner but were not referred to the breast clinic. Of the 69 women reporting breast cysts, 57 (83%) were also seen in an outpatient clinic, and 27 (39%) required further review.

Patients reporting breast pain and tenderness were not regarded as necessarily requiring clinical review, and checking on their clinical management is not a priority task for the research team. However, if the women report severe pain and ask for help or assessment, they are contacted. Furthermore, the hospital records of a sample reporting mastalgia were checked to try to determine patterns of clinical management. A total of 93 women who entered the study in the months January–March, 1980–85, reported breast pain over the previous 12 months. Of these 38 (40%) had attended breast clinic and 10 (11%) required further review. Another 12 women had consulted their general practitioner, but 38 (40%) had not sought medical help for their symptoms.

NON-RESPONDERS

A review of the non-responders amongst the January 1980–85 study entries showed that of the 87 initial non-responders, 45 (51.7%) replied after a reminder. A further six had had an outpatient appointment for a benign breast problem in the past year, and ten had had other hospital treatment. New addresses were found for five study women and general practitioners have confirmed the absence of breast disease in a further seven women. Altogether, 14 required further follow-up, particularly for changes of address. Thus follow-up may be unsatisfactory in 5% of patients.

CONCLUSIONS

In summary, this study gives an overall view of the prevalence of breast symptoms in a population of women with a previous symptomatic referral to a breast clinic for benign problems. A total of 71% of women replied to an annual questionnaire, 17% of whom reported a breast symptom, and 9% attended outpatients for a breast problem over the preceding 12 months. Breast complaints remain extremely common and represent a significant demand on medical resources.

Women responding to the annual breast review have participated in a study of breast cancer risk for 5–10 years. Response rates were similar for all dates of entry to the study, showing that prospective follow-up can be maintained for 10 and more years. Prospective studies of breast cancer risk factors can, in addition, yield considerable information concerning the natural history of benign breast disease.

ACKNOWLEDGEMENT

The research described in this paper is supported by Cancer Research Campaign.

REFERENCE

1. Wolfe, J.N. (1976). Risk of breast cancer development determined by mammographic parenchymal pattern. *Cancer*, **37**, 2486–92

SECTION 2

The normal human breast

12

Overview of the menstrual cycle

M. Elstein

INTRODUCTION

All events occurring in sexually sensitive end-organs in the female are governed by the actions of the sex steroids emanating from the ovary. These tissue responses result from the actions of the ovarian steroids which are mediated by receptor proteins, which are both cellular and nuclear. The anterior pituitary has been termed the 'conductor' of the endocrine 'orchestra' controlling all endocrinal events as well as those affecting the menstrual cycle. However, it is the hypothalamus which serves as the 'director' controlling the actions of the anterior pituitary. The messages from the hypothalamus control the action of the anterior pituitary by means of releasing factors. The hypothalamus itself is controlled by the 'committee' in the form of cerebral centres which are influenced by environmental factors within and outside the body.

The menstrual cycle is therefore manifest by changes not only in the reproductive organs but also in other tissues, as well as the breasts which are the topic of this book. Both the influence of environmental factors from outside the person, and the effects of the endogenous environment are described in this chapter. The changes of the ovarian cycle associated with the fluctuations in ovarian steroids are also presented. These result in bodily changes as well as emotional effects during the menstrual cycle. However, most of the changes of the menstrual cycle manifest in the reproductive organs.

Changes in the reproductive tract, especially its vascularity, are influenced by the human sexual response which in turn also has an important influence on the breast. The response of the breast to sexual stimulation needs to be taken into account in assessing breast changes during the menstrual cycle.

CYCLICITY OF THE MENSTRUAL CYCLE

One of the most important features of the menstrual cycle is its regular pattern, occurring usually every 28 days with the external manifestation of menstrual loss. However, it has been stated that one of the outstanding features of the regularity of the menstrual cycle is its irregularity. Indeed, this irregularity is most manifest in the first 4–6 years after the menarche. The irregularity which extends between 35 and 50 days results usually from the frequent occurrence of anovular cycles, which are common for a while after the onset of menstrual function, i.e. the menarche. Human ovulatory cycles tend to be longer because of the longer duration of the proliferative phase. In the third and fourth decade of a woman's life, the range of the duration of the menstrual cycle diminishes with an average duration of 28–30 days. This is usually associated with regular ovulation and a relatively constant luteal phase of 14 days' duration. In the 4–6 years preceding the menopause, however, women tend to have markedly irregular cycles, with the frequent occurrence of anovular cycles with a mean cycle duration extending to 60, or (if one includes one standard deviation) up to 80 days. This primarily is due to frequent anovular cycles, although an increased duration of the proliferative phase is not an unusual added factor. This has been demonstrated by the work of Treloar[1] (Figure 1).

CONTROL OF THE MENSTRUAL CYCLE

The menstrual cycle is controlled by the secretions of the anterior pituitary. The two gonadotrophins are the follicle stimulating hormone (FSH) and luteinizing hormone (LH). These glycoprotein hormones take their names from their action on the ovary, although they also have an effect on the male. Although 20% of the molecule is carbohydrate, the polypeptide part plays the important endocrine role. Each of these

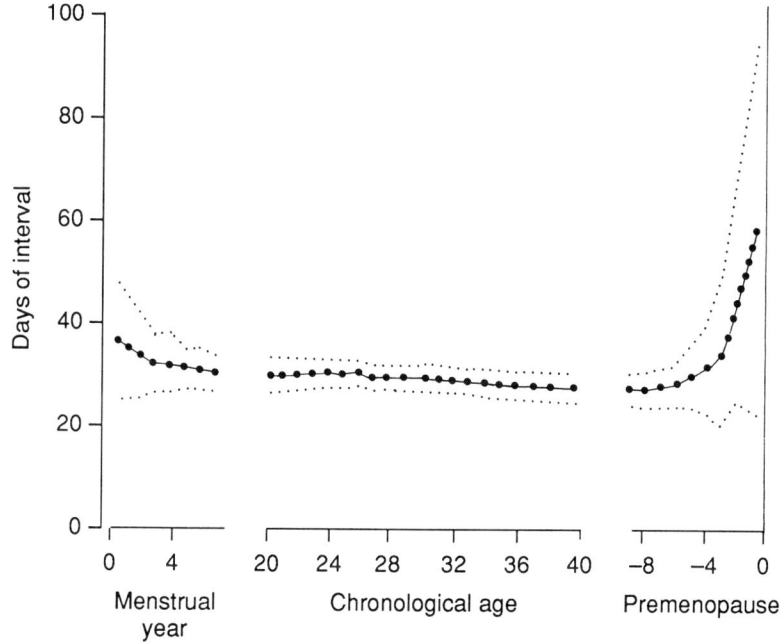

Figure 1 Range of duration of menstrual cycle. Solid line = yearly means, dotted lines = yearly standard deviation[1]

gonadotrophins consists of two sub-units. The α subunit is common to both LH and FSH, but it is the β subunit which carries the specific hormonal activity and it is here that there are differences between LH and FSH. Both these gonadotrophins are synthesized in the same cells of the anterior pituitary but each has its own storage vesicles. There is a circadian rhythm which is clearly identifiable before, and during, puberty in addition to the classic monthly cycle.

The gonadotrophin releasing hormones (GnRH) are small decapeptides which control the release of the gonadotrophins. There is strong evidence that one peptide regulates the secretions of both the gonadotrophins. GnRH is secreted in a pulsatile fashion, controlling the release of the gonadotrophins which consequently also appear in a pulsatile manner.

The gonadotrophins are controlled by a feedback mechanism which operates at three levels:

(1)   A long loop from ovarian steroids;

(2)   A short loop from pituitary gonadotrophins;

(3)   An ultra-short loop from the releasing hormones.

Most of these endocrine feedback loops are negative, although the mid-cycle surge to precipitate ovulation is the result of a positive feedback effect with rising oestrogen resulting in a peak of LH, triggering ovulation at mid-cycle. There is a concomitant lesser peak of FSH.

Throughout the cycle there is a continual tonic release of both these gonadotrophins with an increase in the FSH:LH ratio in the first half of the cycle.

The hypothalamic centres are under the control of cerebral centres or 'bio-clocks'. These serve as a 'pulse generator' to ensure that the GnRH neurons function in a synchronous manner. From the GnRH centres in the hypothalamus, the GnRH polypeptides are released in pulses, which occur every 90 minutes, into the hypothalamic pituitary portal system. These hypothalamic centres are controlled by a complex network of neural interactions which are influenced by various stimuli and which reach extra-hypothalamic structures as a result of the external environment. It is no surprise, therefore, that emotional factors can control the menstrual cycle as well as other physiological events (Figure 2).

EXTERNAL INFLUENCES AFFECTING PITUITARY–OVARIAN FUNCTION

The two major sensory exteroceptive stimuli which most profoundly influence reproductive function are light and duration of day length and olfaction, as perceived by pheromones.

Light

There is good evidence that light and sleep influence gonadotrophin activity and especially LH output and its pulsatility in humans. It is believed that these influences are mediated by the pineal gland, most

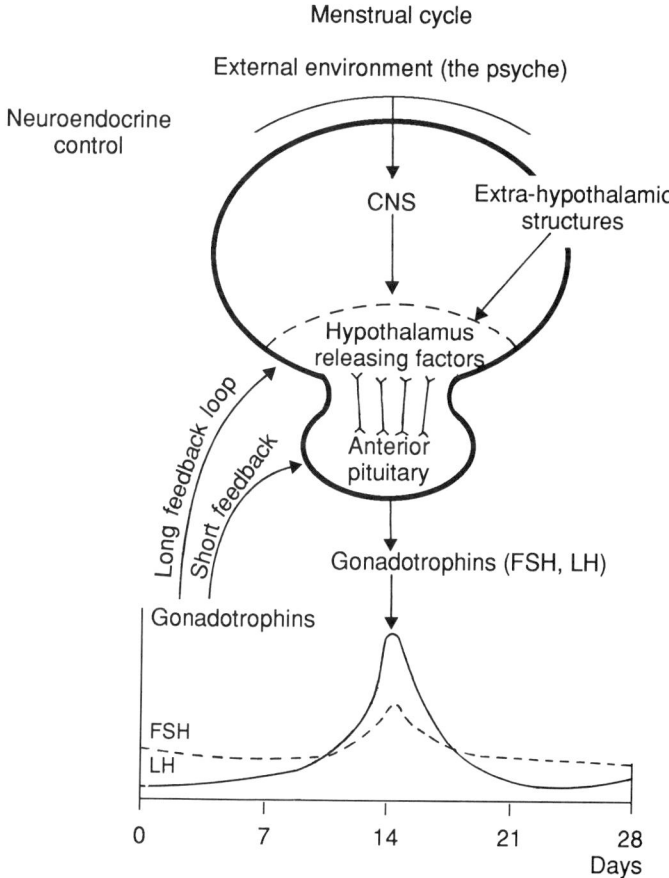

Figure 2 Central nervous influences on pituitary function

evidence for this being available from animal data (especially sheep) rather than that for humans. It is well established that melatonin levels are very low during the day and increase dramatically at night and, more importantly, that melatonin secretion is related to daylight length. Seasonal influences on reproductive function, in particular the inhibition of sexual function during the dark winters of the Arctic North, have been well documented, although seasonal influences in human beings have been modified by the artificial environment that man has developed around him. Nevertheless, the pineal gland would appear to be the mechanism through which light stimuli are mediated by the output and rhythm of melatonin secretion.

Blindness is associated with a precocious menarche. Girls who are blind experience the menarche 7 months earlier, on average, than non-blind controls. It is possible, therefore, that the stimulus afforded by light is inhibitory to human sexual maturation. Its absence could therefore be a factor in advancing pubertal development, hence the hypothesis of the inhibition of the reproductive system by the pulsatile secretion of melatonin from the pineal gland which is influenced by the amount of light the subject receives.

Smell

The possibility that reproductive function might be influenced by an olfactory mechanism, mediated by pheromones, has a firmer basis than that of the influence of light. It is well known that sexual function in animals can be stimulated by olfactory sensory mechanisms. Perfumes are not the only evidence to support the hypothesis that pheromones influence human sexual behaviour. It is well known that menstrual cycles of girls become synchronized with close contact[3].

Additionally, there are male-derived pheromones which exert an influence on the menstrual cycle and the incidence of ovulation. It appears that proximity to males exerts a significant influence on the woman's menstrual cycle.

EXERCISE-ASSOCIATED MENSTRUAL DYSFUNCTION

Pubertal development and the menarche are commonly delayed in competitive athletes and ballet dancers. Additionally, women who partake of vigorous exercise have a higher prevalence of secondary amenorrhoea. The mechanism for this inhibition of pituitary–ovarian function seems to be more related to the stress of the training, rather that to any psychological factors. Contributing to this effect is the fact that these women often have low body-fat stores and have been subjected to weight loss during their training. However, it would be naive to consider that the decrease in body fat is the prime factor in the genesis of this suppression of pituitary–ovarian function. It is possible that there are a number of mechanisms operating and that stress *per se* may be of major significance with the reproductive suppression being the manner in which conservation of energy, that might otherwise be expended by the reproductive processes, could be achieved.

This stress- and exercise-related suppression of hypothalamic–pituitary function, resulting in amenorrhoea and menstrual disturbance, is associated with reduction in body fat. The questions arise whether this is a causal relationship, whether the suppression of the hypothalamus is a reflection of poor nutrition, as often occurs in these women, or whether this is a result of the intense training process.

FAT STORES

A woman's reproductive cycle may be profoundly influenced by changes in her nutritional status. The confounding effects of voluntary weight reduction and exercise on the mechanism by which nutrition and hence fat stores could influence pituitary function are difficult to elucidate. The relationship between lean, very fit women and their high activity and physical exertion on hypothalamo–pituitary function and what factor is due to dietary restriction, cannot readily be identified.

However, a useful example of the adaptive process in nature is shown by the i'Kung women, who only ovulate when food is plentiful. These women store fat in their lower body, demonstrate a lower body segmental obesity and tend to have little disturbance of reproductive function.

Conversely, obesity associated with impaired reproductive function, and in particular an excess of androgen production, demonstrate an upper body segment obesity. These women manifest a higher incidence of menstrual dysfunction and abnormal carbohydrate metabolism. They have also recently been shown to be more prone to breast malignancy. If this observation is substantiated, the practice of treating benign breast disease with androgens might well have to be reconsidered.

THE OVARIAN CYCLE

The influences outlined above control the ovarian cycle, which in turn releases fluctuating levels of ovarian steroids which manifest in changes in the endocrine-sensitive end-organs. The human fetus receives its quota of primary oocytes during intrauterine life. During childhood there is some follicular growth without maturation. There is a marked reduction in oocytes from just under five million, less than 1/20th of that number surviving puberty. Nevertheless, with each monthly cycle 20 or more follicles will begin to develop and one or two dominant follicles take over to be stimulated to achieve ovulation. Following ovulation, there is an invasion of the follicle with theca interna cells and vessels and a transformation of the granulosa cells to form the corpus luteum of the cycle.

During the proliferative or follicular phase there is a rapidly increasing secretion of oestrogens which reaches a peak, coinciding with the maximal size of the dominant follicle. This triggers a positive feedback on the hypothalamus and the pituitary to cause a peak release of LH, resulting in ovulation within 36–48 hours. The final growth of the primary follicle, once established, appears to be independent of pituitary stimulation. The corpus luteum produces progesterone and oestrogens, reaching its maximal action if pregnancy occurs. Otherwise it degenerates and atrophies 10 days after ovulation.

Changes in the ovarian cycle can be monitored serially by the non-invasive ultrasound method, which allows a clear and precise tracking of the developing follicle during the menstrual cycle.

GENERAL BODY CHANGES DURING THE MENSTRUAL CYCLE

During the menstrual cycle, with fluctuating ovarian steroids, there is a tendency for an increase in fluid retention and weight gain during the luteal phase as a result of the influence of progesterone with oestrogen. There is a slowing of bowel motility, with a tendency to constipation, and predisposition to allergic conditions worsens[4].

CHANGES IN THE GENITAL TRACT

Endometrium

The ovarian steroids and their changing levels are directly reflected by the changes in the endometrium which occur at different stages of the menstrual cycle. The endometrium comprises two layers, a basal and a functional. The latter is divided into a spongy and compact layer, the latter being more superficial. The cyclic changes affect all components of the endometrium, i.e. the glands, stroma and vessels. The endometrium is richly vascularized. There are classic histological criteria for dating of the endometrium[5].

Cervix

The functions of the cervix are mediated by its mucus which manifests a number of rheologically related properties, including viscosity, spinnbarkeit, flow elasticity or retraction, elasticity and tack[6]. During the menstrual cycle at the time of oestrogen dominance, cervical mucus is watery and thin with the maximal spinnbarkeit associated with optimal sperm penetrability. At that time, mucus shows a ferning phenomenon. The cervical canal is patulous with a cascade of thin watery mucus. These changes can be used as a bioassay of oestrogenic action on the cervical epithelium and have clinical application. Following ovulation, the cervical mucus becomes thickened, opaque and viscid and impenetrable to sperm.

Vaginal cytology

The vaginal epithelium is a stratified squamous epithelium in which the mature superficial cells have pyknotic nuclei. Under oestrogen dominance, the desquamated vaginal squamous cells are flattened, discrete, with small nuclei with a clean surrounding area containing no debris. After ovulation the epithelial cells are desquamated from a deeper level in the epithelium and have larger nuclei showing their chromatin pattern. Their edges are curled up and the cells tend to clump together. This progesterone effect was previously used as an indicator of progesterone activity. This application has now been superseded by blood hormone assays.

PSYCHOLOGICAL MANIFESTATION OF THE MENSTRUAL CYCLE

There are distinctive changes in women's affect and mood during the menstrual cycle which modify sensory perception. At the time of oestrogen dominance, awareness of pain is diminished and pain thresholds are elevated. At this time there is heightened awareness, and visual and acoustic ability is enhanced. Other sensory functions are also at their optimum including the perception of touch, taste and olfaction. Susceptibility to sexual arousal is at its peak during the time of ovulation when there is oestrogen dominance, and also recurs during the latter part of the luteal phase[4]. Indeed, at the time of the preovulatory oestrogen surge, the woman will often initiate sexual activity. She will have a feeling of well-being, assertiveness and maximum creativity at this time.

MORBID PSYCHOLOGICAL BEHAVIOUR

There are major differences in the data concerning the incidence of women who complain of premenstrual and perimenstrual malaise and poor function. Cross-cultural studies illustrate a marked divergence in the manifestation of the so-called premenstrual syndrome. There is little doubt that such a syndrome exists where women have morbid thoughts and a higher level of depression and anxiety in the premenstrual phase. Some women manifest changes of mood and may even complain of uncontrolled behaviour patterns and aggressiveness. There are other somatic manifestations of the premenstrual syndrome such as fluid retention and breast discomfort. The condition popularly known as 'PMT' is probably a conglomerate of different symptom complexes associated with biochemical changes in susceptible women, as a result of the endocrine pattern of the menstrual or dysfunctional menstrual pattern. The precise mechanisms of these abnormalities are unknown. It is well established, however, that women manifesting psychopathic behaviour often present at the time of the premenstrual and menstrual phases such as in rates of hospitalization for psychiatric indications, suicidal attempts and disorderly behaviour patterns in institutionalized females. In the normal population there is an increased susceptibility to accidents and behaviour disturbances during this time.

HUMAN SEXUAL RESPONSE AND THE BREAST

It is not generally appreciated by general surgeons that the breast is a sexually responsive organ and manifests vasocongestion with increase in size following sexual arousal. This often results in erection of the nipples and engorgement of the areolar glands. The breast's vasocongestion with resulting enlargement occurs more often in breasts which have not lactated. The breasts will undergo a cycle of vasocongestion similar to the pelvic organs, with a subsequent detumescence of the sexually aroused and congested tissues. This vasocongestion and relaxation is often independent of the pelvic vascular changes. Continued vascular congestion may result in pain and discomfort in the breasts.

CONCLUSION

This brief overview of the dynamic changes in female endocrinology during the menstrual cycle concerns the physical manifestations as well as emotional effects on women, in addition to the genital tract changes which have been well documented. These systemic and emotional effects are influenced by environmental and cultural factors, many of which remain obscure. Moreover, the human sexual response cycle results in vascular congestion and is usually followed by relaxation of this congestion. Disturbances of function can result in persistent congestion which, in the case of the breast, can be a confounding factor in the management of breast symptoms.

REFERENCES

1. Treloar, A.E., Boynton, R.E., Behn, B.G. and Brown, B.W. (1967). Variation of the human menstrual cycle through reproductive life. *Int. J. Fertil.*, **12**, 77–126
2. van Vogt, D.A. (1990). Influences of the visual and olfactory systems on reproduction. *Sem. Reprod. Endocrinol.*, **8**, 1–14
3. McClintock, M.K. (1971). Menstrual synchrony and suppression. *Nature (London)*, **229**, 244–5
4. Asso, D. (1983). *The Real Menstrual Cycle.* (Chichester: John Wiley and Sons Ltd)
5. Noyes, R.W., Hertig, A.T. and Rock, J. (1950). Dating the endometrial biopsy. *Fertil. Steril.*, **1**, 3
6. Elstein, M. (1978). The structure and function of cervical mucus. *Br. Med. Bull.*, **34**, 83–5

13

Heterogeneity in the stromal components of the mammary gland: relevance to the development of breast disease

A.M. Schor, S.L. Schor, J.E. Ferguson, G. Rushton, A. Howell and M.W.G. Ferguson

EPITHELIAL–STROMAL INTERACTIONS IN THE MAMMARY GLAND

The central role played by the stroma in the morphogenesis of the mammary gland during embryonic development was demonstrated a number of years ago by Kratochwil[1]. In heterotypic recombination studies involving the co-culture of embryonic epithelium with salivary mesenchyme, the mammary epithelial tissue was observed to form salivary-like tubular structures. In addition to this abnormal pattern of branching morphogenesis, mammary epithelial cells also began to invade into the adjacent salivary mesenchyme. In contrast, both salivary and mammary epithelia, co-cultured with their respective mesenchymes, underwent organ-specific morphogenesis and remained completely circumscribed, showing no evidence of invasive behaviour. These results raise the interesting possibility that a phenotypic characteristic generally associated with neoplastic transformation, i.e. local invasion into the surrounding stroma, may be expressed by *normal* epithelial cells when they are in contact with an *atypical* stroma.

The mammary epithelial stalk of the male mouse embryo begins to degenerate at day 15 of gestation; this programmed epithelial cell death occurs in response to testosterone produced by the developing testes, and is preceded by the formation of a dense condensation of mesenchyme around the primitive mammary stalk. Durenberger and colleagues[2] demonstrated that the primary target of testosterone is the mammary mesenchyme and that this tissue must first be made 'competent' by interaction with the invading mammary epithelial stalk. Identical results regarding the important role of the mesenchyme in mediating the effects of testosterone on the pattern of prostate epithelial cell differentiation have been reported by Cunha[3].

Fibroblasts are the principal cell type present in the stroma. A number of co-culture studies have revealed that the presence of fibroblasts is required for mammary epithelial cells to exhibit appropriate steroid responsiveness *in vitro*. For example, oestrogen was reported to have no effect on mammary epithelial cells cultured on their own, whilst the addition of oestrogen to co-cultures of murine mammary epithelial cells and fibroblasts resulted in epithelial cell proliferation and synthesis of progesterone receptors[4,5]. The oestrogen induction of epithelial cell proliferation depended on the direct contact of epithelial cells with fibroblasts, whereas the induction of progesterone receptor did not; this induction also occurred in the presence of fibroblast-conditioned medium, as well as when the epithelial cells were cultured in a substratum of type I collagen. This latter observation is of particular relevance regarding the nature of the signalling mechanisms operative between epithelial cells and fibroblasts *in vitro*; in certain situations direct cell–cell contact is required (a condition that would not occur in normal tissues *in vivo*), whilst in other situations soluble products and insoluble matrix components produced by fibroblasts appear to be effective signalling agents.

Numerous studies have revealed that ubiquitous matrix macromolecules produced by fibroblasts, such as collagen and proteoglycans, exert a profound effect upon the proliferation, migration, differentiation and morphogenesis of mammary epithelial cells[6–11]. The manner in which interaction with macromolecular constituents of the extracellular matrix affects these diverse aspects of epithelial cell behaviour is not understood in detail, but appears to be related to alterations in cell shape[11].

In addition to matrix molecules, fibroblasts produce a number of soluble factors which function as paracrine regulators of neighbouring epithelial cell behaviour[12–14]. The biological activity of these soluble factors (cytokines) and the nature of the extracellular matrix in contact with epithelial cells are mutually interdependent in the sense that, firstly, cytokines tend to be pleiotropic effectors, influencing various aspects of cell behaviour, including matrix deposition, and, secondly, cellular responsiveness to cytokines is modulated by the nature of the extracellular matrix upon which they are growing[15].

Signalling between epithelium and stroma is not unidirectional. The epithelium has been shown to exert a profound effect upon various aspects of fibroblast function, including matrix deposition, and the secretion of matrix degrading enzymes[6-19]. The nature of this 'dynamic reciprocity', whereby epithelium and stroma influence each other in a self-regulating fashion, has been reviewed by Bissell and colleagues[20].

CHANGES IN THE EXTRACELLULAR MATRIX OF THE NORMAL BREAST DURING THE MENSTRUAL CYCLE

The functional unit of the normal human breast – 'the lobule' or 'terminal duct–lobular unit' – is composed of glandular epithelial ductules surrounded by a specialized connective tissue called the intralobular stroma. This stroma contains numerous fibroblasts embedded within a relatively loose extracellular matrix. Lobules are separated from each other by a dense connective tissue, the interlobular stroma, which contains a more sparse population of fibroblasts. Specific changes in the appearance and composition of the intralobular stroma have been reported to occur in synchrony with the secretion of ovarian steroid hormones during the menstrual cycle[21-24]. These changes were not observed in the interlobular stroma, suggesting that interactions between epithelium and intralobular fibroblasts may be important in determining epithelial response to hormones and growth factors.

We have recently documented changes in the distribution of various macromolecular constitutents of the extracellar matrix in the normal breast during the menstrual cycle[25,26]. In this study, normal breast biopsies were obtained from 31 women undergoing surgery for benign fibroadenoma or reduction mammoplasty. The age, final histological diagnosis and day of the menstrual cycle were recorded. Immunostaining with a panel of polyclonal antibodies to matrix macromolecules was performed and the pattern of staining in the following compartments was then analysed: ductular basement membrane, sub-basement membrane zone, delimiting layer of fibroblasts, intralobular stroma and interlobular stroma. Our results have revealed the following results:

(1) The intensity of staining for laminin, type IV collagen and heparan sulphate proteoglycan in the basement membrane changed during the cycle: maximal staining for all of these components occurred during weeks 1 and 4 and was significantly reduced during weeks 2 and 3, thus implying a co-ordinate control in their deposition.

(2) The staining of tenascin in the basement membrane displayed a different pattern; namely, this macromolecule was more abundant in the basement membrane during the last 2 weeks of the cycle. Other matrix macromolecules present in the basement membrane (e.g. type VI collagen) remained unchanged during the menstrual cycle.

(3) Surprisingly, molecules generally considered to be confined to the basement membrane (i.e. type IV collagen and laminin) were also observed in the sub-basement membrane zone, delimiting layer of fibroblasts and intralobular stroma.

(4) Significant changes occurred during the cycle in the staining pattern of fibronectin in the intralobular stroma: maximal staining was observed during weeks 1 and 4, whereas staining was significantly reduced during weeks 2 and 3.

It should be noted that the basement membrane of blood vessels, although containing the same extracellular matrix molecules as the ductular basement membrane, showed no changes during the cycle. Our results suggest that the variations observed in the ductules during the menstrual cycle reflect hormonally-induced changes in extracellular matrix synthesis and/or degradation.

The existence of hormonally-regulated changes in the extracellular membrane has important implications for tumour pathologists, utilizing immunoflourescent antibodies to basement membrane components (e.g. laminin and type IV collagen) to distinguish between the intact basement membrane of carcinoma *in situ* and the interrupted basement membrane diagnostic of microinvasive disease. As this study has demonstrated a major reduction and even absence of certain basement membrane components during weeks 2 and 3 of the normal menstrual cycle, errors in distinguishing between carcinoma *in situ* and microinvasive disease may be made at this time in the cycle, when the amount of certain extracellular constituents is normally low. Although it is not known whether such cyclic regulation also occurs in carcinoma *in situ*, possible errors in diagnosis could be minimized by confining biopsies to weeks 1 and 4 of the menstrual cycle, when the expression of exracellular matrix components of the normal basement membrane is maximal.

EPITHELIAL–STROMAL INTERACTIONS INFLUENCE THE BEHAVIOUR OF MAMMARY CARCINOMA CELLS

Paradoxically, mammary carcinoma cells are considerably more difficult to culture on their own than normal epithelial cells. Indeed, investigators working in this field have commonly observed that the majority of cells which survive and which may be subcultured from primary breast tumours are normal cells rather than the expected neoplastic population[27] (our own observations and numerous personal communications). The preferential growth of tumour cells has, however, been observed in co-cultures with specific types of fibroblasts[28], including those of fetal origin[29].

As is the case with normal epithelial cells, interactions between neoplastic epithelial cells and stromal cells are mediated both by matrix macromolecules and soluble factors. For example, the growth of mammary carcinoma cells is enhanced by culture on type I collagen substrata, as well as the more complex extracellular matrices deposited by endothelial cells and fibroblasts[30–32]. Further evidence has indicated that carcinoma cells grown on three-dimensional collagen matrices exhibit an *in vivo*-like response to cytotoxic drugs[33]. Soluble factors produced by breast fibroblasts have been reported to stimulate markedly the proliferation of mammary carcinoma cells[34]. Carcinoma cells exert a reciprocal stimulatory effect upon the proliferation of stromal fibroblasts, again mediated by the secretion of soluble factors[35,36] and deposition of matrix macromolecules[37]. The invasive and metastatic potential of tumour cells has been related to the production of matrix degrading enzymes[38,39]. The production of these enzymes by stromal fibroblasts is significantly stimulated by interaction with neoplastic cells[40,41].

FUNCTIONAL HETEROGENEITY AMONGST FIBROBLASTS AND ITS IMPLICATIONS FOR EPITHELIAL–STROMAL INTERACTIONS

Various lines of evidence indicate that fibroblasts display a considerable degree of functional heterogeneity. For example, fetal fibroblasts differ from their normal adult counterparts in a number of respects, including the production of soluble growth and migration stimulating factors[15,42–44] and matrix macromolecules[45]. Fetal-to-adult transitions in these phenotypic characteristics occur at various times during normal development and are believed to play a central role in the control of inductive epithelial–stromal interactions[46]. More recently, extensive functional heterogeneity has been observed within the fibroblasts of a given tissue (reviewed in reference 15). This *intra*-site heterogeneity of fibroblasts may play an important role in tumour progression and metastasis. Tumour-derived fibroblasts have been reported to release higher levels of collagenolytic activity than normal fibroblasts and were more responsive to stimulation by tumour-conditioned medium[47]; these authors conclude that host fibroblasts appear to be a heterogeneous population of responsive and non-responsive cells with respect to interaction with tumour cells. It has also been shown that lactogenic hormones lead to the synthesis of casein by mouse epithelial cells only if co-cultured with two particular sublines of 3T3 fibroblasts[48]; Swiss 3T3 and human fibroblasts were not effective.

In view of the important role played by fibroblasts in signalling epithelial cell behaviour, it is not surprising that aberrant fibroblasts have been implicated in the pathogenesis of cancer. Cancer patient fibroblasts exhibit a number of behavioural and biochemical abnormalities commonly associated with transformation, such as the ability to form colonies in semi-solid medium, reduced serum requirement for growth and prolonged lifespan *in vitro* (reviewed in ref. 15).

Our own work in this area has demonstrated that fibroblasts plated onto the surface of collagen gel substrata migrate down into the underlying three-dimensional macromolecular matrix at rates which are dependent upon a number of experimental parameters, including cell density[49]. At any given time after plating, the percentage of cells present within the gel may be ascertained by simple microscopic observation[50]. Using this experimental approach, we initially reported that confluent fetal fibroblasts migrate into three-dimensional collagen gels to a significantly greater extent than do their normal adult counterparts. We subsequently reported:

(1) Tumour-derived fibroblasts obtained from approximately 50% of sporadic breast cancer patients expressed a fetal-like migratory phenotype[51];

(2) Skin fibroblasts obtained from the same patients also exhibited fetal-like migratory behaviour, thus indicating the systemic nature of this stromal cell abnormality[51,52];

(3) Skin fibroblasts obtained from greater than 90% of patients with familial breast cancer similarly behaved in a fetal-like fashion[53].

The unaffected first-degree relatives of familial breast cancer patients are at a greatly elevated lifetime risk of developing breast cancer themselves; it is, therefore, of interest that skin fibroblasts obtained from approximately 50% of such individuals displayed fetal-like behaviour[54]. Skin fibroblasts obtained from patients with a wide variety of other types of tumours of epithelial and mesenchymal origin were also demonstrated to display a fetal-like mode of migratory behaviour[52].

These differences in migratory behaviour have subsequently been shown to result from the production of a soluble 'migration stimulating factor' (MSF) by fetal fibroblasts and the fetal-like fibroblasts of cancer patients[55]; in contrast, normal adult fibroblasts do not produce MSF, but retain responsiveness to it, thus providing a convenient bioassay for this factor. MSF has now been purified to homogeneity[56]. Initial biochemical characterization indicates that it has a molecular mass of approximately 70 kDa, binds to heparin with moderate affinity, is cationic and has an unusually high content of proline (13.3 residues per 100). MSF differs from other recently described motility factors, e.g. scatter factor[44,57] and autocrine motility factor[58], in terms of various biochemical parameters and target cell specificities.

Hyaluronate is a major biosynthetic product of fibroblasts and has been shown to affect a number of cellular processes of potential relevance to tumour development, including cell migration, differentiation and angiogenesis. We have recently reported that MSF exerts a direct stimulatory effect upon hyaluronic acid synthesis by a target adult fibroblast line[59], thus suggesting one possible mechanism whereby its inappropriate production by aberrant (fetal-like) fibroblasts in the adult might contribute to cancer pathogenesis.

Fetal fibroblast cultures *in vitro* undergo a spontaneous transition to a characteristically adult-like mode of migratory behaviour after 50–55 population doublings, i.e. approximately three-quarters of their *in vitro* lifespan[60]. We have demonstrated that this acquisition of an adult migratory phenotype results from a concomitant cessation in MSF production[55].

On the basis of the above observations, we have put forward the following hypothesis suggesting a direct involvement of fetal-like fibroblasts in cancer pathogenesis[61,62]:

(1) Fetal fibroblasts undergo a programmed cessation in MSF production during the course of normal development which is manifest *in vitro* by the acquisition of an adult migratory phenotype.

(2) This transition does not occur in certain individuals.

(3) The persistent expression of fetal phenotypic characteristics by fibroblasts in these individuals puts them at an elevated risk of developing cancer, most probably as a result of a dysfunction in normal epithelial–mesenchymal interactions.

Experimental support of this hypothesis has been provided by Sakakura[63] who observed that implantation of fetal (but not adult) fibroblasts into the adult rat mammary gland induced the hyperplastic growth of the normal epithelial elements and rendered these more sensitive to overt transformation by carcinogenic agents.

Recent observations have indicated that serum obtained from 88% (23/26) of cancer patients contained detectable levels of MSF, whereas such activity was found in the serum of only 10% (2/20) of healthy controls[64]. The quantitative assessment of serum MSF levels may, therefore, provide a means for identifying individuals in the population at elevated risk of developing cancer.

FIBROBLAST HETEROGENEITY IN THE NORMAL MAMMARY GLAND

Samples of breast tissue have been obtained from patients undergoing surgery for benign lesions, carcinoma of the breast and reduction mammoplasty. These tissues were digested with collagenase and hyaluronidase. Using differential incubation times and sedimentation, we have been able to isolate four fibroblast populations from normal breast samples; these populations have been named Fractions I, II, III and IV. Fraction I represents the fibroblasts that separate first from the tissue, once the fat has been removed, and are presumed to be derived from the interlobular stroma. Fraction IV represents the fibroblasts closest to the epithelial cells, often growing out of epithelial organoids and are, consequently, presumed to derive from the intralobular stroma. Fractions II and III are intermediate; Fraction II is most likely to be similar to Fraction I and Fraction III similar to Fraction IV. It should be emphasized that this division into Fractions I–IV is based on the isolation technique used. Proof that these Fractions represent at least two different populations comes from the *in vitro* characterization that we have carried out (see below).

A preliminary characterization has been carried out with 20 normal breast fibroblast lines which represent the interlobular (Fraction I) and intralobular (Fraction IV) fibroblasts from ten patients. Five of these patients had carcinoma of the breast, but no signs of lesion in the 'normal breast tissue' used to obtain the fibroblasts. The remaining five patients had either reduction mammoplasty or fibroadenoma.

Our results (unpublished) demonstrated that all interlobular fibroblasts were fetal-like regarding their migratory phenotype and the presence of migration-stimulating activity in their conditioned medium. In contrast, intralobular fibroblasts were adult-like when obtained from non-tumour patients but fetal-like when derived from the 'normal breast' of carcinoma patients.

With the caveat of the small number of lines studied, our results suggest that normal interlobular fibroblasts are fetal-like regarding their migratory phenotype and the production of MSF, whereas normal intralobular fibroblasts (as well as skin fibroblasts[55]) are adult-like. This difference between interlobular and intralobular fibroblasts appears to be lost in the 'normal breast' of carcinoma patients; in five specimens examined both interlobular and intralobular fibroblasts were fetal-like in their migratory behaviour but still differed from each other by other criteria, such as response to transforming growth factor β and cytokine production (unpublished results). Whether these aberrant fibroblasts precede (and possibly promote) the development of an epithelial lesion is not known. However, in the light of our current knowledge of epithelial–stromal interactions, it is likely that the presence of fetal-like fibroblasts adjacent to the lobular epithelium may disrupt normal epithelial function and facilitate its migration and proliferation.

REFERENCES

1. Kratochwil, K. (1969). Organ specificity in mesenchymal induction demonstrated in the embryonic development of the mammary gland of the mouse. *Dev. Biol.*, **20**, 46–71
2. Durenberger, H., Heuberger, B., Schwartz, P., Wasner, G. and Kratochwil, K. (1978). Mesenchyme-mediated effect of testosterone on embryonic mammary epithelium. *Cancer Res.*, **38**, 4066–70
3. Cunha, G.R. (1984). Androgenic effects upon prostatic epithelium are mediated via trophic influences from stroma. In Kimball, F.A., Buhl, A.E. and Carter, D.B. (eds.) *Progress in Clinical and Biological Research*, Vol. 145, *New Approaches to the Study of Benign Prostatic Hyperplasia*, pp. 81–102. (New York: Alan R. Liss)
4. McGrath, C.M. (1983). Augmentation of the response of normal mammary epithelial cells to estradiol by mammary stroma. *Cancer Res.*, **43**, 1355–60
5. Haslam, S.Z. (1986). Mammary fibroblasts influence on normal mouse mammary epithelial cell responses to estrogen *in vitro*. *Cancer Res.*, **46**, 310–16
6. Richards, J., Pasco, D., Yang, J., Guzman, R. and Nandi, S. (1983). Comparison of the growth of normal and neoplastic mouse mammary cells on plastic, on collagen gels and in collagen gels. *Exp. Cell. Res.*, **146**, 1–14
7. McGrath, M., Palmer, S. and Nandi, S. (1985). Differential response of normal rat mammary epithelial cells to mammogenic hormones and EGF. *J. Cell. Physiol.*, **125**, 182–91
8. Li, M.L., Aggeler, J., Farson, D.A., Hatier, C., Hassell, J. and Bissell, M.J. (1987). Influence of reconstituted basement membrane and its components on casein gene expression and secretion on mouse mammary epithelial

cells. *Proc. Natl. Acad. Sci. USA*, **84**, 136-40

9. Parry, G., Cullen, B., Kaetzel, C.S., Kramer, R. and Moss, L. (1987). Regulation of differentiation and polarized secretion in mammary epithelial cells maintained in culture: extracellular matrix and membrane polarity influences. *J. Cell. Biol.*, **105**, 2043-3051

10. Park, C.S. and Bissell, M.J. (1986). Messenger RNA for basement membrane components in the mouse mammary gland and in cells in culture. *J. Cell. Biol.*, **103** abstr. 380, 101a

11. Streuli, C.H. and Bissell, M.S. (1990). Expression of extracellular matrix components is regulated by substratum. *J. Cell. Biol.*, **110**, 1405-15

12. Lawrence, D.A., Pircher, C.K.M. and Jullien, P. (1984). Normal embryo fibroblasts release transforming growth factor in latent form. *J. Cell. Physiol.*, **121**, 184-8

13. Oka, T., Kurachi, H., Yoshimura, M., Tsutsumi, O., Cossu, M.F. and Saga, M. (1987). Study of the growth factors for the mammary gland; epidermal growth factor and mesenchyme-derived growth factors. *Nucl. Med. Biol.*, **14**, 353-60

14. Sporn, M.B. and Roberts, A.B. (1986). Peptide growth factors and inflammation, tissue repair and cancer. *J. Clin. Invest.*, **78**, 329-32

15. Schor, S.L. and Schor, A.M. (1987). Clonal heterogeneity in fibroblast phenotype: implications for the control of epithelial–mesenchymal interactions. *Bio. Essays*, **76**, 200-4

16. Johnson-Wint, B. and Gross, J. (1984). Regulation of connective tissue collagenase production: stimulators from adult and foetal epidermal cells. *J. Cell. Biol.*, **98**, 90-6

17. Iozzo, R.V. (1985). Neoplastic modulation of the extracellular matrix. *J. Biol. Chem.*, **260**, 7464-73

18. Vanio, D., Jalkanen, M. and Thesleff, I. (1989). Syndecan and tenascin expression is induced by epithelial mesenchymal interactions in embryonic tooth mesenchyme. *J. Cell. Biol.*, **108**, 1945-54

19. Simon-Assman, P., Bouziges, F., Arnold, C., Haffen, K. and Kedinger, M. (1988). Epithelial and mesenchymal interactions in the production of basement membrane components in the gut. *Development*, **102**, 339-47

20. Bissell, M.G. and Barcellos-Hoff, M.H. (1987). The influence of the extracellular matrix on gene expression: is structure the message? *J. Cell Sci.*, Suppl. 8, 327-43

21. Ozello, L. and Speer, F.D. (1958). The mucopolysaccharides in the normal and diseased breast. Their distribution and significance. *Am. J. Pathol.*, **34**, 993-1009

22. Ozello, L. (1970). Epithelial–stromal junction of normal and dysplastic mammary glands. *Cancer*, **23**, 586-600

23. Fanger, H. and Ree, J.H. (1974). Cyclic changes of human mammary gland in relation to the menstrual cycle. An ultrastructural study. *Cancer*, **34**, 574–85

24. Eyden, B.P., Watson, R.J., Harris, M. and Howell, A. (1986). Intralobular fibroblasts in the resting human mammary gland: ultrastructural properties and intercellular relationships. *J. Submicrosc. Cytol.*, **18**, 397–408

25. Ferguson, J.E., Schor, A.M., Howell, A. and Ferguson, M.W.J. (1990). The distribution of tenascin in the normal breast during the menstrual cycle and in carcinoma. *Differentiation*, **42**, 199–207

26. Ferguson, J.E., Schor, A.M., Howell, A. and Ferguson, M.W.J. (1991). Chances in the extracellular matrix of the normal human breast during the menstrual cycle. *Cell Tissue Res.*, submitted for publication

27. Buehring, G.C. and Williams, R.R. (1976). Growth rates of normal and abnormal human mammary epithelia in cell culture. *Cancer Res*, **36**, 3742–7

28. Zipori, D., Krupsky, M. and Resnitzky, P. (1987). Stromal cell effects on clonal growth of tumours. *Cancer*, **60**, 1757–62

29. Armstrong, R.C. and Rosenau, W. (1978). Cocultivation of human primary breast carcinomas and embryonic mesenchyme resulting in the growth and maintenance of tumour cells. *Cancer Res.*, **38**, 894–900

30. Stampfer, M., Hallowes, R.C. and Hackett, A.J. (1980). Growth of normal mammary cells in culture. *In Vitro*, **16**, 415–25

31. Fridman, A., Alon, Y., Doljanski, F., Fuks, Z. and Vlodavsky, I. (1985). Cell interaction with the extracellular matrices produced by endothelial cells and fibroblasts. *Exp. Cell. Res.*, **158**, 461–76

32. Biran, S., Vlodavsky, I., Fuks, Z., Lijovetzsky, G. and Horowitz, A.T. (1986). Growth of human mammary carcinoma cells from biopsy specimens in serum-free medium on extracellular matrix. *Int. J. Cancer*, **38**, 345–54

33. Vescio, R.A., Redfern, C.H., Nelton, T.J., Uroretz, S., Stern, P.H. and Hoffman, R.M. (1987). *In vivo*-like responses of human tumours growing in three-dimensional gel-supported primary culture. *Proc. Natl. Acad. Sci. USA*, **84**, 5029–33

34. Enami, J., Enami, S. and Koga, M. (1983). Growth of normal and neoplastic mouse mammary epithelial cells in primary culture: stimulation by conditioned medium from mouse mammary fibroblasts. *Gann*, **74**, 845–53

35. Peres, R., Betshotz, C., Westermark, B. and Heldin, C.H. (1987). Frequent expression of growth factors for mesenchymal cells in mammary carcinoma cell lines. *Cancer Res.*, **47**, 3425–9

36. Barsky, S.H. and Gopalakrishna, R. (1987). Isolation of a myofibroblast

growth factor from human carcinoma cell lines *Biochem. Biophys. Res. Commun.*, **149**, 1125–31

37. Kao, R.T., Hall, J., Engel, L. and Stern, R. (1984). The matrix of human breast tumour cells is mitogenic for fibroblasts. *Am. J. Pathol.*, **115**, 109–16

38. Liotta, L.A., Rao, C.N. and Barsky, S.H. (1983). Tumour invasion and the extracellular matrix. *Lab. Invest.*, **49**, 636–49

39. Moscatelli, D. and Rifkin, D.B. (1988). Membrane and matrix localisation of proteinases: a common theme in tumour cell invasion and angiogenesis. *Biochim. Biophys. Acta*, **948**, 67–85

40. Dabbous, M.K., El-Torky, M., Haney, L., Brinkley, B. and Sobhy, N. (1983). Collagenase activity in rabbit carcinoma: cell source and cell interactions. *Int. J. Cancer*, **31**, 357–64

41. Biswas, C. and Toole, B.P. (1987). Modulation of the extracellular matrix by tumour cell-fibroblast interactions. In Elson, E., Frazier, W. and Glaser, L. (eds.) *Cell Membranes, Methods and Reviews*, Vol. 3, pp. 341–63. (New York: Plenum Press)

42. Clemmons, D.R. (1983). Age-dependent production of a competence factor by human fibroblasts. *J. Cell. Physiol.*, **114**, 61–7

43. Stoker, M. and Perryman, M. (1985). An epithelial scatter factor released by embryo fibroblasts. *J. Cell. Sci.*, **77**, 209–24

44. Stoker, M., Gherardi, E., Perryman, M. and Gray, J. (1987). Scatter factor is a fibroblast derived modulator of epithelial cell mobility. *Nature (London)*, **327**, 239–42

45. Matsura, H. and Hakomori, S.I. (1985). The oncofetal domain of fibronectin defined by a monoclonal antibody FDC-6: its presence in foetal and tumour tissues and its absence in those from normal tissue and plasma. *Proc. Natl. Acad. Sci, USA*, **83**, 6517–21

46. Caplan, A.I., Fiszman, M.Y. and Eppenburger, H.M. (1983). Molecular and cell isoforms during development. *Science*, **221**, 921–7

47. Dabbous, M.K., Haney, L., Carter, L.M., Paul, A.K. and Reger, J. (1987). Heterogeneity in fibroblast response to host-tumour cell–cell interactions in metastatic tumours. *J. Cell. Biochem.*, **35**, 333–44

48. Levine, J.F. and Stockdale, F.E. (1985). Cell–cell interactions promote mammary epithelial cell differentiation. *J. Cell. Sci.*, **100**, 1415–22

49. Schor, S.L., Schor, A.M., Winn, B. and Rushton, G. (1982). The use of three dimensional collagen gels for the study of tumour cell invasion *in vitro*: experimental parameters influencing cell migration into the gel matrix. *Int. J. Cancer*, **29**, 57–62

50. Schor, S.L. (1980). Cell proliferation and migration of collagen substrata *in vitro*. *J. Cell. Sci.*, **41**, 159–75

51. Durning, P., Schor, S.L. and Sellwood, R.A.S. (1984). Fibroblasts from patients with breast cancer show abnormal migratory behaviour *in vitro*. *Lancet*, **1**, 890–2

52. Schor, S.L., Schor, A.M., Durning, P. and Rushton, G. (1985). Skin fibroblasts obtained from cancer patients display foetal-like migratory behaviour on collagen gels. *J. Cell. Sci.*, **73**, 235–44

53. Schor, S.L., Haggie, J.A., Durning, P., Howell, A., Smith, L., Sellwood, R.A.S. and Crowther, D. (1986). Occurrence of a fetal fibroblast phenotype in familial breast cancer. *Int. J. Cancer.*, **37**, 831–6

54. Haggie, J., Howell, A., Sellwod, R.A., Birch, J.M. and Schor, S.L. (1987). Fibroblasts from relatives of patients with hereditary breast cancer show fetal-like behaviour *in vitro*. *Lancet*, **1**, 1455–7

55. Schor, S.L., Schor, A.M., Grey, A.M. and Rushton, G. (1988). Foetal and cancer patient fibroblasts produce an autocrine migration stimulating factor not made by normal adult cells. *J. Cell. Sci.*, **90**, 391–9

56. Grey, A.M., Schor, A.M., Rushton, G., Ellis, I. and Schor, S.L. (1989). Purification of the migration stimulating factor produced by foetal and breast cancer patient fibroblasts. *Proc. Natl. Acad. Sci. USA*, **86**, 2438–42

57. Gherardi, E., Gray, J., Stoker, M., Perryman, M. and Furlong, R. (1989). Purification of scatter factor; a fibroblast-derived basic protein that modulates epithelial interactions and movement. *Proc. Natl. Acad. Sci. USA*, **86**, 5844–8

58. Liotta, L.A., Mandler, R., Murano, G., Katz, D.A., Gordon, R.K., Chiang, P.K. and Schiffman, E. (1986). Tumour cell autocrine motility factor. *Proc. Natl. Acad. Sci. USA*, **83**, 3302–6

59. Schor, S.L., Schor, A.M., Grey, A.M., Chen, J., Rushton, G., Grant, M.E. and Ellis, I. (1989). Mechanism of action of the migration stimulating factor (MSF) produced by foetal and cancer patient fibroblasts: effect on hyaluronic acid synthesis. *In Vitro Cell. Develop. Biol.*, **25**, 737–46

60. Schor, S.L., Schor, A.M., Rushton, G. and Smith, L. (1985). Adult, foetal and transformed fibroblasts display different migratory phenotypes on collagen gels: evidence for an isoformic transition during foetal development. *J. Cell. Sci.*, **73**, 221–34

61. Schor, S.L., Schor, A.M., Howell, A. and Crowther, D. (1987). Hypothesis: persistent expression of foetal phenotypic characteristics by fibroblasts is associated with an increased susceptibility to neoplastic disease. *Exp. Cell. Biol.*, **55**, 11–17

62. Schor, S.L., Schor, A.M., Howell, A. and Haggie, J.A. (1987). The possible role of abnormal fibroblasts in the pathogenesis of breast cancer. In Rich, M.A., Hager, J.C., and Lopez, D.M. (eds.) *Breast Cancer: Scientific and*

Clinical Progress, pp. 142–57. (Lancaster: Kluwer Academic Publishers)
63. Sakakura, T. (1983). Epithelial–mesenchymal interactions in mammary gland development and its pertubation in relation to tumorigenesis. In Rich, M.A., Hager, J.C. and Furmanski, P. *Understanding Breast Cancer*, pp. 261–84. (eds.) (New York: Marcel Dekker)
64. Picardo, M., Schor, S.L., Schor, A.M. and Howell, A. (1990). The presence of migration stimulating factor (MSF) in the serum of breast cancer patients. *Lancet*, **337**, 130–3

14

The proliferation of normal human breast tissue in nude mice is stimulated by oestrogen and not progesterone

I.J. Laidlaw, R. Clarke, E. Anderson, A.W.M.C. Owen, C.S. Potten and A. Howell

INTRODUCTION

Epidemiological evidence indicates that the risk of breast cancer is related to the hormonal pattern of premenopausal women with cyclic production of large amounts of oestrogen and progesterone[1,2]. This hormonal profile causes a greater increase in risk than the pattern in postmenopausal women – constant low oestrogen with very low progesterone – but gives no indication of the relative importance of these two ovarian hormones[3]. Biopsy studies of the human breast show clearly that proliferation of the breast is lowest in the follicular phase of the menstrual cycle and highest in the luteal phase, with a peak between 21 and 25 days[4,5]. Studies of the proliferation of human breast xenografts in nude mice determined that oestrogen was the major mitogen for the stimulation of DNA synthesis, with progesterone alone having a minor stimulatory effect[6]. The doses of steroid hormone given were not examined but were said to be physiological on the basis that a stimulatory effect was observed. No explanation of the dose of progesterone was given. Stimulation of primary cultures of breast epithelial cells with supraphysiological doses of oestrogen and progesterone showed oestrogen alone to be stimulatory with progesterone having no effect[7]. At physiological levels, synthetic progestogens inhibit the mitogenic action of oestrogen in these systems[8]. By contrast, biopsy studies of endometrial cell division show maximal proliferation in response to low levels of oestrogen in the early follicular phase and that, in the luteal phase, in the presence of progesterone there is virtually no proliferation[9], the progesterone secretion having a dramatic antiproliferation effect. There are two commonly held explanations of the hormonal control of breast epithelia. The first is that oestrogen in the follicular phase induces some proliferative activity then the addition of progesterone, secreted in the luteal phase, initiates a much greater proliferative response. Laboratory studies have not demonstrated such a major proliferative response to progesterone. The alternative hypothesis is that oestrogen alone induces breast cell division with little or no modification by progesterone. This requires that there be a dose–response relationship between proliferation and the serum oestrogen in the range found in the human menstrual cycle and that the induced change is delayed between 4 and 5 days from initiation of the stimulus.

Knowledge of the hormonal factors which stimulate proliferation of the normal breast and modulate their effects through alteration in receptor expression may help elucidate the mechanisms of both initiation and promotion. This, in turn, may lead to the development of preventive treatments for those at high risk and formulations of contraceptives and hormone replacement therapy with a theoretically lower risk of breast cancer[10,11].

MATERIALS AND METHODS

Patients

One hundred and nineteen samples of breast tissue were obtained from 87 females presenting for surgery to remove a clinically isolated lesion of the breast. None of the patients had a history of either carcinoma (invasive or *in situ*) or diffuse breast disease. The majority ($n = 82$) were solitary fibroadenomas; histology of the remainder showed no abnormality ($n = 3$), epidermoid cyst ($n = 1$) and mammary duct ectasia ($n = 1$).

Athymic nude mice

All the animals used were intact 8–10-week-old adult female athymic nude mice BALB/c (*nu/nu*) obtained from our own colony, housed in flexible-fill isolators (Bantin and Kingman, Hull, UK), which provided a sterile environment by utilizing high-efficiency particulate air filters. During the period of experiments they were kept in isolators (North Kent Plastics Ltd, Dorset, Kent), and given sterilized irradiated (5 Mrads) feed. Autoclaved water and bedding were used throughout. Surgical procedures were performed under sterile conditions with halothane inhalation anaesthesia (Halovet Vapouriser 8% version).

Hormone treatment of nude mice

The methods for administration and assessment of exogenous oestrogen and progesterone were similar. Normal serum levels of oestrogen and progesterone for adult nude mice were established by radioimmunoassay of mouse serum. A number of silastic implants delivering oestrogen or progesterone were tested. The serum steroid levels obtained were estimated at the conclusion of each experimental group in the majority of treated mice.

Samples of breast tissue were taken at least 1 cm from the clinically abnormal area and only tissue showing no macroscopic abnormality was sampled. This tissue was divided into several portions under sterile conditions and eight portions of approximate size $2 \times 1 \times 1$ mm were transplanted to the nude mice. A small portion of each sample was divided into 1 mm strips and incubated immediately in tritiated thymidine ($1\,\mu$Ci/ml), for 1 h at $37°$C. These were fixed in Carnoys' solution until processed for autoradiography.

At least 1000 epithelial cells per specimen were counted. Areas for counting were selected out of focus at low power, then complete high-power fields were counted between two or more of the sections. The number of labelled cells was expressed as a percentage of the total number of cells counted. A cell was considered labelled when five or more silver grains were seen overlying an epithelial cell. In the vast majority of cases the grain count considerably exceeded this number.

The xenografts were sampled 14, 21, 28 and in some instances 35 days after implantation. A silastic pellet bearing the additional steroid was implanted after the sample at 14 days had been removed, but during the same procedure. A group of mice had no additional steroid. Oestrogen was given by means of four pellet sizes bearing 0.5, 1.0, 2.0 or 6.0 mg of oestradiol. Progesterone was given as either 4.0 or 8.0 mg pellets. One group of mice received oestrogen 2.0 mg, then an additional pellet bearing progesterone 4.0 mg was implanted a week later to allow combined therapy.

Statistical methods

The Friedman test, which is a two-way analysis of variance by ranks for matched samples, testing whether three or more samples are from the same population, was used for the preliminary analysis of the labelling indices. If this test proved significant at the level of 5% or less, the differences between groups was tested with the Wilcoxon signed rank test, using a reduced significance level of 0.05 divided by the number of tests.

RESULTS

Normal human breast tissue was obtained from 103 women, mean age $27.4 \pm$ SD 7.2 years. Ovarian steroid levels were maintained at appropriate human luteal phase levels in the mice with the 2 mg oestradiol pellet (oestradiol, 800–1500 pmol/l) and 4.0 mg progesterone pellet (progesterone, 38–54 nmol/l). Lobular architecture was maintained for at least 56 days in untreated animals. The thymidine labelling index (TLI) fell from its initial value (median and interquartile range = 1.46%, 0.95–2.29, $n = 68$) to a nadir by 14 days after implantation (median and interquartile range = 0.49%, 0.20–0.68, $n = 39$) and remained low at 28 (median and interquartile range = 0.41%, 0.19–0.67, $n = 39$) and 56 days (median and interquartile range = 0.41%, 0.28–0.75, $n = 42$) (Figure 1). This decrease was statistically significant (Friedman's, $p = 0.0001$). Administration of the 2 mg pellet of oestrogen from the 14th day induced a statistically significant rise in the TLI (median and interquartile range, day $21 = 2.10\%$, 1.39–2.96, $n = 43$; day $28 = 2.53\%$, 1.81–3.04, $n = 40$; Friedman's, $p = 0.0001$) (Figure 2). Sampling xenografts at daily intervals after implantation of the 2.0 mg oestrogen pellet showed there was an incremental response to oestrogen after an initial lag of 3 days. While this appeared to be a progressive

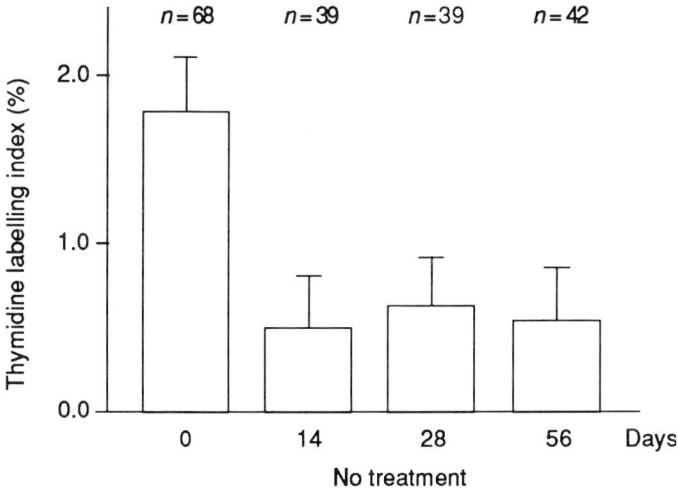

Figure 1 The thymidine labelling index in relation to the day of sampling. The mice were not treated with exogenous steroid. There was a highly significant difference in the TLI (Friedman's, $p = 0.0001$) on comparing untreated xenografts (days 14, 21 and 28) with the TLI determined in the patient sample (day 0, Wilcoxon sign rank, $p \leq 0.002$). There were no further significant differences between the TLI observed after 1 or 2 weeks

rise and overall was statistically significant (Friedman's, $p = 0.0001$), no differences could be demonstrated between any of the individual groups (Wilcoxon signed rank tests were not significant at stringency ≤ 0.001388; Figure 3). Assessment of the response to incremental doses of oestrogen was undertaken. Although there was a progressive increase in TLI to incremental oestrogen, this was not statistically significant (Friedman's, not significant; Figure 4). Neither 7 nor 14 days progesterone treatment increased the TLI above the untreated control values (median and interquartile range, day $14 = 0.48\%$, $0.20–0.70$, $n = 39$; day $21 = 0.54\%$, $0.32–0.80$, $n = 36$; day $28 = 0.50\%$, $0.36–0.88$, $n = 38$: Friedman's, not significant; Figure 5). The TLI after combined oestrogen and progesterone for 2 weeks was median and interquartile range, day $35 = 1.63\%$, $1.39–1.95$, $n = 30$, compared with median and interquartile range, day $35 = 1.86\%$, $1.59–2.16$, $n = 43$ for

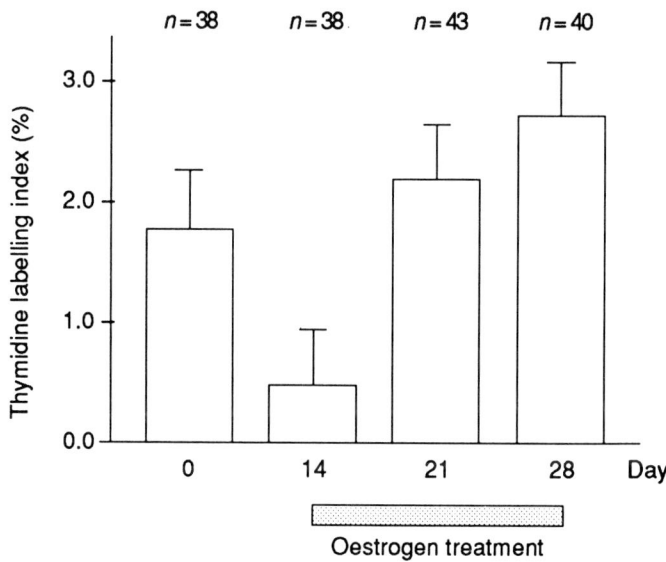

Figure 2 The thymidine labelling index in relation to the day of sampling. The mice were implanted with a silastic pellet bearing 2 mg of oestrogen on day 14 after the xenografts for that time had been removed. There was a highly significant difference in the TLI (Friedman's, $p = 0.0001$) and on comparing untreated xenografts (day 14) and the TLI determined in both the patient sample (day 0, Wilcoxon sign rank) and the TLI in the oestrogen-treated xenografts (days 21 and 28). There was no significant difference between the TLI observed after 1 or 2 weeks of oestrogen

oestrogen treatment alone (Mann–Whitney U test, not significant; Figure 6).

DISCUSSION

The tissue utilized for these studies was histologically normal breast taken from adult women with a fibroadenoma. These lesions are well circumscribed and are found in otherwise normal breasts, and other related studies have used tissue derived from the same source[4,7,12]. The data show that the proliferative activity of these normal breasts, as

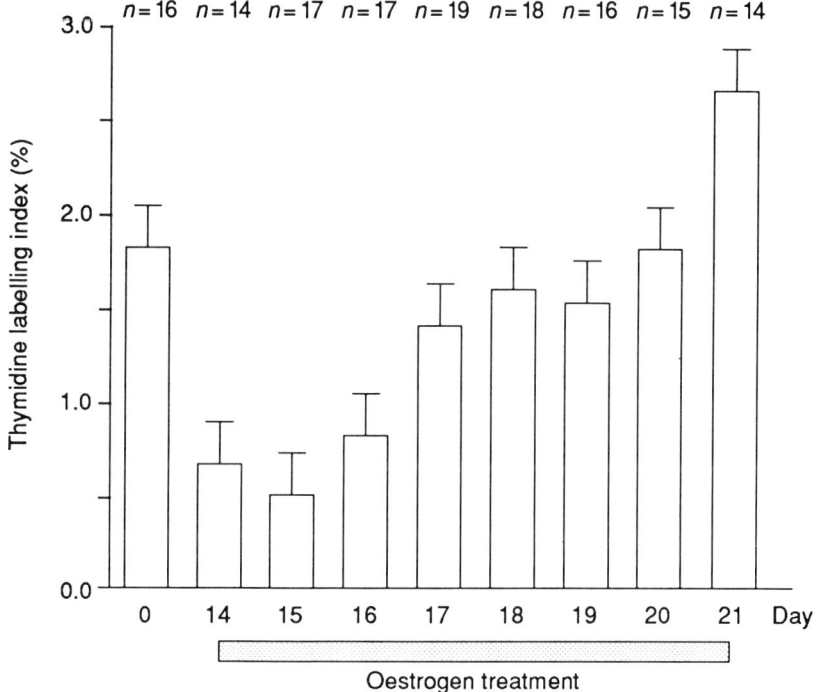

Figure 3 The onset of proliferation after implantation of the silastic pellet bearing 2 mg of oestradiol. There was a significant trend in the TLI after the onset of the stimulus (Friedman's test, $p = 0.0001$)

measured by the thymidine labelling index (TLI), was in keeping with that found by other observers[7].

There was considerable variability in the TLI both between patients and within a patient. Technical errors in the preparation of autoradiographs and counting errors contribute to a proportion of the remaining variability, but this and previous studies using identical techniques indicate that these are small, implying that other biological factors must account for the differences[7].

The finding, in this model, that oestrogen alone stimulated epithelial proliferation within the normal physiological range for oestrogen in a dose-related fashion is strong evidence that this hormone is the major mitogen for normal human breast epithelium. The serum level of oestrogen in the untreated animals approximated to that of postmeno-

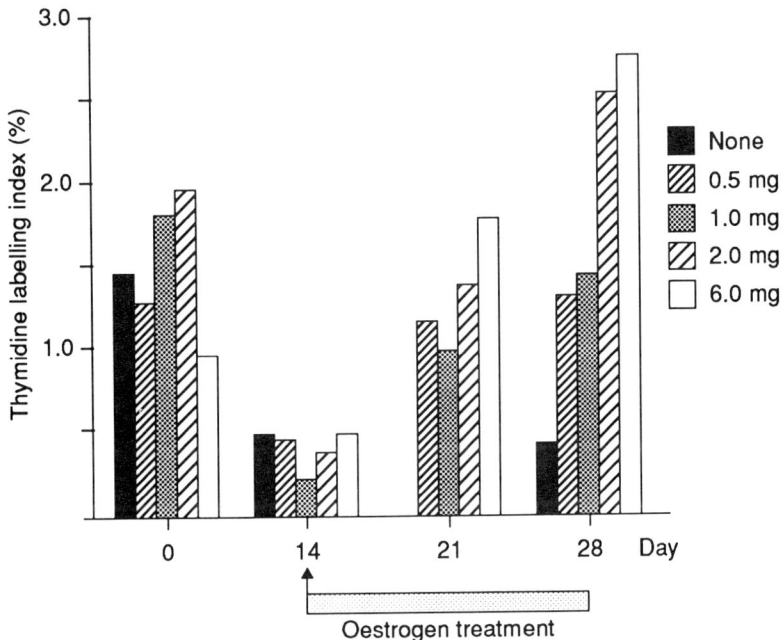

Figure 4 The thymidine labelling index in relation to the dose of oestrogen administered. The mice were implanted with a silastic pellet bearing either 0.5, 1.0, 2.0 or 6.0 mg of oestrogen on day 14 after the xenografts for that time had been removed. All the samples were then taken after 1 week's treatment. The composite histogram shows the TLI (median) observed in xenografts from both the untreated and oestrogen-treated xenografts when resampled at 21 and 28 days. There was no statistically significant trend associating dose of oestrogen with the TLI observed at either day 21 or day 28

pausal women, who are also deficient in progesterone. In this hormonal environment the level of proliferation in the xenografts was close to the activity observed in these older women *in vivo*[12]. The median TLI stimulated by oestrogen closely approximated that observed in the patients who contributed this tissue, suggesting this is the maximum level possible for this tissue, thereby reinforcing that a physiological level of oestrogen is a competent stimulus for normal breast epithelial turnover. No evidence of a proliferative response to progesterone was observed in the xenografts exposed to either a physiological or supraphysiological level of progesterone in the absence of oestrogen.

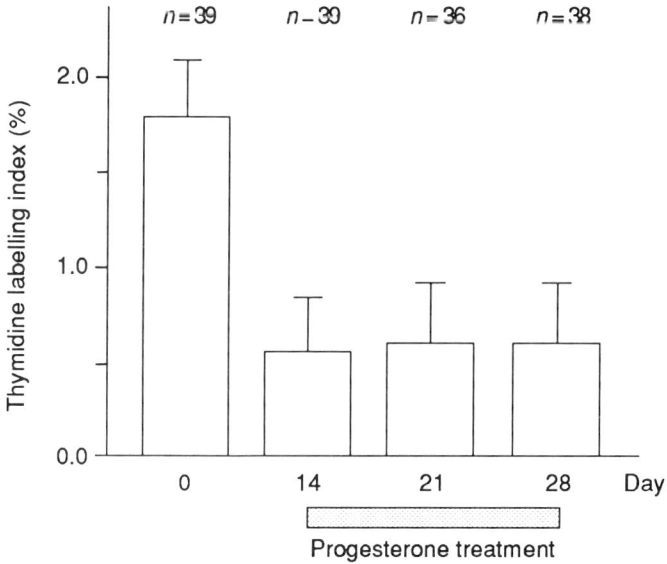

Figure 5 The thymidine labelling index in relation to the day of sampling. The mice were implanted with a silastic pellet bearing 4 mg of progesterone on day 14 after the xenografts for that time had been removed. There was a highly significant difference in the TLI (Friedman's, $p = 0.0001$). Comparing the TLI obtained from untreated xenografts (day 14) and the TLI determined in the progesterone-treated xenografts (days 21 and 28) showed no significant differences. The TLI at any of these points was significantly lower than that in the patient samples

This would have been difficult to demonstrate given the number of samples and the low level of proliferation in the untreated samples. There was no statistical difference between the TLI in grafts stimulated by oestrogen and progesterone and those treated with oestrogen alone.

The combined oral contraceptive pill has been associated with an increased incidence of breast cancer and both the oestrogen and progesterone activities of these preparations have been linked to the risk[13]. Some studies have shown that the early occurrence of regular cycles is associated with an increased risk of breast cancer[14,15]. Regular cycles are more likely to be ovulatory and therefore associated with progesterone secretion. These authors suggest that progesterone is the determinant of proliferation, albeit on a background of oestrogen secretion, and that this progesterone-driven division is of import in the increased risk associated with the pill. This contradicts the earlier

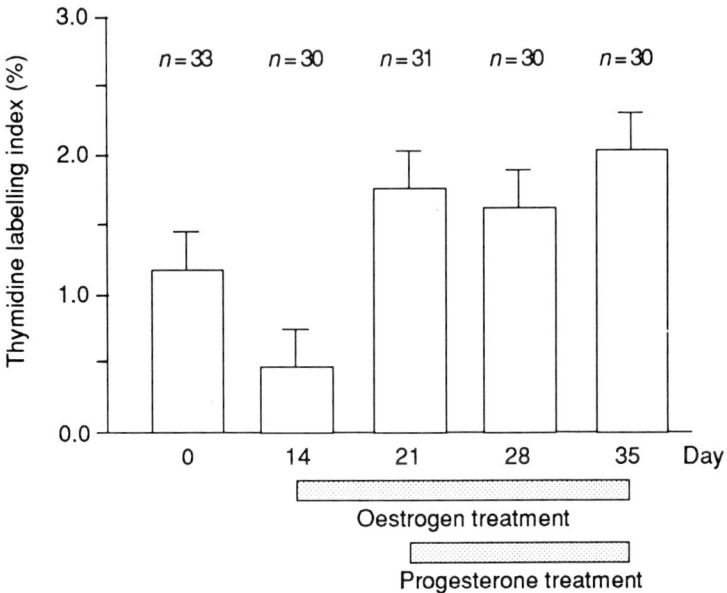

Figure 6 The thymidine labelling index (TLI%; median and 75th percentile) in relation to the day of sampling. The mice were treated with 2 mg of oestrogen from day 14 and 4 mg of progesterone from day 21 (Friedman's test, $p = 0.0001$). Comparisons of the TLI from the patient sample (day 0) with the TLI in the xenografts treated with oestrogen alone on day 21, or combined oestrogen and progesterone on days 28 and 35 at the reduced significance level of 0.005 (Wilcoxon signed-rank test) were not significant and further there was no statistically significant difference observed between the TLI observed in any of the treated xenografts. The TLI in the untreated xenografts (day 14) was significantly lower than the TLI determined in the patient sample (Wilcoxon signed-rank test: day 0 vs. day 14, $p = 0.0001$) and the TLI in the xenografts treated for 1, 2 or 3 weeks (Wilcoxon signed-rank test: day 0 vs. day 21, $p = 0.3173$; day 0 vs. day 28, $p = 0.4155$; day 0 vs. day 35, $p = 0.1747$)

'oestrogen window' hypothesis that early cycles were anovulatory, which provided the breasts with an uninterrupted oestrogen stimulation, which was associated with an increased risk of breast cancer[16]. However, competent cycles are associated with much higher luteal phase levels of oestrogen than anovulatory cycles, so if progesterone has little or no effect on proliferation then ovulatory cycles might also be expected to have an increased stimulatory effect. In these studies no evidence of a proliferative response to progesterone was found, whereas a direct relationship was identified between the oestrogen stimulus and breast epithelial proliferation.

If lobuloepithelial proliferation is related to an increased risk of breast cancer, then this study supports the hypothesis that oestrogen rather than progesterone is of major importance in the human.

ACKNOWLEDGEMENTS

The authors would like to thank all the clinical and secretarial staff at the breast clinic for their assistance in many ways throughout the period of this study.

REFERENCES

1. Lillienfield, A.M. (1956). Relationship of cancer of the female breast to artificial menopause and marital status. *Cancer*, **9**, 927–34
2. Feinleib, M. (1968). Breast cancer and artificial menopause; a cohort study. *J. Natl. Cancer Inst.*, **41**, 315–29
3. Henderson, B.E., Ross, R.K., Judd, H.C., Krailo, M.D. and Pike, M.C. (1985). Do regular cycles increase breast cancer risk? *Cancer*, **56**, 1206–8
4. Going, J.J., Anderson, T.J., Battersby, S. and MacIntyre, C.C.A. (1988). Proliferative and secretory activity in human breast during natural and artificial menstrual cycles. *Am. J. Pathol.*, **130**, 193–203
5. Potten, C.S., Watson, R.J. and Williams, G.T. (1988). Cell proliferation in the normal human breast. The effect of age and menstrual cycle upon proliferative activity of the normal human breast. *Br. J. Cancer*, **58**, 163–70
6. McManus, M.J. and Welsch, C.W. (1984). The effect of estrogen, progesterone, thyroxine, and human placental lactogen in DNA synthesis of human breast ductal epithelium maintained in athymic nude mice. *Cancer*, **54**, 1920–7
7. Longman, S.M. and Buehring, G.C. (1987). Oral contraceptives and breast cancer. *In vitro* effect of contraceptive steroids on human mammary cell growth. *Cancer*, **59**, 281–7
8. Mauvais-Jarvis, P., Kuttenn, F. and Goupel, A. (1986). Antioestrogen action of progesterone in breast tissue. *Breast Cancer Res. Treatment*, **8**, 179–87

9. Ferenczy, A., Bertrand, G. and Gelfand, M.M. (1979). Biopsy studies of the proliferation of human endometrium. *Am. J. Obstet. Gynecol.*, **133**, 859–67

10. Fentimann, I.S. (1990). *Detection and Treatment of Early Breast Cancer*, pp. 252–62. (London: Dunitz)

11. Pike, M.C., Ross, R.K. and Lobo, R.A. (1990). LHRH agonists and the prevention of breast and ovarian cancer. *Br. J. Cancer*, **60**, 142–5

12. Anderson, T.J., Ferguson, D.J.P. and Raob, G.M. (1982). Cell turnover in the resting breast; influence of parity, contraceptive pill, age and laterality. *Br. J. Cancer*, **46**, 376–82

13. Anderson, T.J. and Battersby, S. (1989). The involvement of oestrogen in the development and function of the normal breast: histological evidence. In Beck, J.S. (ed.) *Oestrogen and the Human Breast*, pp. 23–34. Proceedings of The Society of Edinburgh

14. Pike, M.C., Henderson, M.C., Krailo, M.D., Duke, A. and Roy, S. (1983). Breast cancer in young women and use of oral contraceptives. Possible modifying effect of formulation and age at use. *Lancet*, **1**, 926–9

15. LaVecchia, C., Decarli, A., DiPietro, S., Francheschi, S., Negri, E. and Parazzini, F. (1985). Menstrual cycle patterns and the risk of breast disease. *Eur. J. Cancer Clin. Oncol.*, **21**, 417–22

16. Korenman, S.G. (1980). Oestrogen window hypothesis of the aetiology of cancer. *Lancet*, **1**, 700–1

15

Functional measures of cyclical changes

S. Battersby, T.J. Anderson, R.J.B. King and K. Mcpherson

BACKGROUND

A number of factors involved in normal breast function have been assessed in relation to the menstrual cycle. These include markers of differentiation, such as α-lactalbumin and cell death (apoptosis), but most attention has focused on proliferation. It is now established that proliferative activity in the 'resting' breast shows variation with the phase of the menstrual cycle, with peak activity in the last week[1,2]. In addition, we have previously highlighted several other parameters influencing proliferation (listed in Table 1)[1]. The important issue remains regarding the question of what are the major factors modulating the proliferative response? Naturally the steroid hormones oestrogen and

Table 1 Independent variables affecting thymidine labelling index (TLI) in breast epithelium

Variable	Effect on TLI
Phase of menstrual cycle	increased in second half
Time since menarche	increased in younger age group
Oral contraceptive use	increased only for nulliparous women
Oral contraceptive composition	increased with oestrogen dose from < 35 to 30–50 μg per day

progesterone have been implicated in its regulation, but there has been some controversy as to their relative importance. In an attempt to clarify their role in breast modulation, we have performed immunohisto-chemical analysis, using monoclonal antibodies to the oestrogen (Abbott) and progesterone (Transbio) receptors.

RESULTS

The study utilized 158 samples of normal breast, obtained from benign breast biopsies, collected as described in an earlier publication[1]. Receptor staining was always nuclear and epithelial predominantly of luminal cells. Cases were scored either on a positive/negative basis or assigned a receptor score, derived as described previously[3]. The effect of phase of the menstrual cycle on receptor reactivity was considered, together with two other influencing variables, oral contraceptive use and parity.

Influence of natural menstrual cycle phase

In the natural menstrual cycle, oestrogen receptor staining was seen in 48% of cases with scores ranging from 0 to 513, median 0. Significantly fewer positive cases were present in the second half of the menstrual cycle, which confirms previous reports and is consistent with down-regulation of oestrogen receptor by progesterone (or possibly oestrogen). Oestrogen receptor showed an inverse correlation with proliferation measured by [³H]thymidine uptake. Progesterone receptor staining was present in 73% of cases, with scores ranging from 0 to 600, median 200. Unlike the endometrial epithelium[4], no relationship was seen with the phase of the cycle and there was no evidence of down-regulation by progesterone or of a relationship with proliferative activity.

Oestrogen and progesterone receptors were not detected in stromal fibroblasts or vascular cells, although proliferation in fibroblasts showed a relationship with menstrual cycle phase, in both natural and oral contraceptive cycles (Figure 1). Uptake of [³H]thymidine by fibroblasts showed greatest frequency on days 21–28 of the cycle, but was also high on days 1–5. Proliferative activity was significantly reduced on days 6–13 compared with days 21–28.

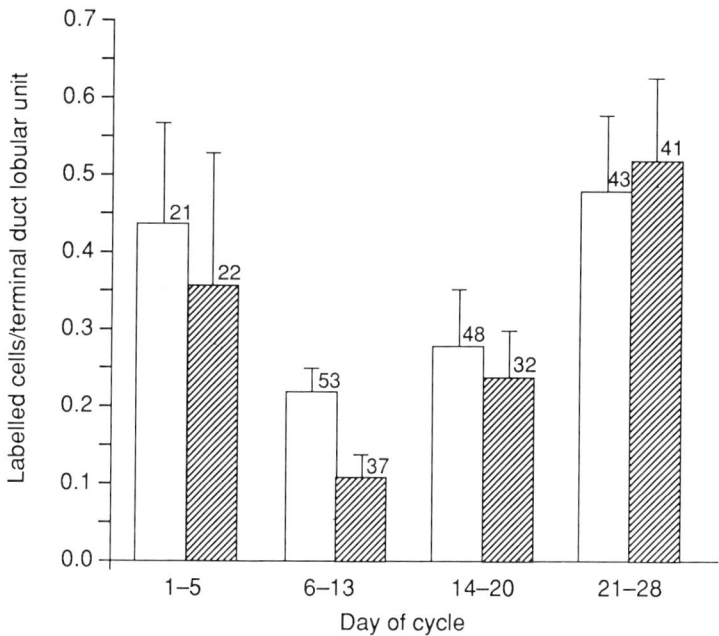

Figure 1 Fibroblast proliferation, measured as the number of [³H]thymidine-labelled cells per terminal duct lobular unit, across natural (empty bars) and oral contraceptive (hatched bars) cycles. Number of cases indicated on bars (16 terminal duct lobular units/case)

Influence of oral contraceptive use

Oestrogen receptor was detected in significantly fewer samples of breast tissue from the oral contraceptive cycle (26%) compared with the natural cycle. This is consistent with receptor down-regulation by progestins. In contrast, progesterone receptor was seen with frequency equal to the natural cycle and, in addition, the median receptor score increased significantly in the second half of the oral contraceptive cycle, suggesting a possible delayed and/or sustained oestrogenic effect in this group.

Influence of parity

No significant differences in steroid receptor staining were seen on comparing tissues taken from parous and nulliparous breasts. However,

Table 2 Independent variables affecting steroid receptor detection in breast epithelium

Variable	Effect on receptor detection
Phase of menstrual cycle	oestrogen receptor decreased in second half
Oral contraceptive use	oestrogen receptor decreased
Interval since last pregnancy	
< 5 years	oestrogen receptor decreased
	progestogen receptor decreased
≥ 5 years	oestrogen receptor increased

it has been noted that breast lobular unit morphology and tissue oestrogen levels may be altered for up to 5 years postpartum. Therefore for parous women in the natural cycle, cases were divided into those pregnant within 5 years and those whose last pregnancy was 5 or more years previously. Comparing these groups, frequency of oestrogen and progesterone receptor positivity showed significant differences. Multivariate analysis allowed consideration of these differences (Table 2) and showed that the likelihood of both oestrogen and progesterone receptor positivity was significantly decreased amongst those recently parous compared with nulliparous. Furthermore, oestrogen receptor showed a highly significant increase amongst those with 5 or more years postpartum, compared with nulliparous. These results suggest a lack of responsiveness or altered local hormonal environment in the lobular units of the breast following pregnancy.

CONCLUSIONS

Evidence from xenograft studies suggests that oestrogen has a direct dose-related effect on proliferation in breast (see Chapter 10). In addition, oestrogen receptor down-regulation in the second half of the cycle is similar to that in the uterus[4] and suggests progesterone responsiveness in breast tissue. However, whilst oestrogen receptor detection in endometrium has a close temporal relationship with proliferation, and the oestrogen effect on breast explants in nude mice occurs in 3 days (see Chapter 10), in breast *in vivo* there is a considerable time delay between evidence of oestrogen action and the peak of proliferative activity. This is true both for natural and oral contraceptive cycles. These results suggest an indirect or delayed effect of oestrogen on proliferation *in vivo*. Further studies are required to resolve the apparent anomalies between the findings obtained *in vitro* and *in vivo*.

The peak proliferation response in breast is seen in the progestogenic phase of the menstrual cycle. This, together with the lack of progesterone receptor down-regulation in the second half of the cycle and during oral contraceptive use, indicates that breast tissue is unlike endometrium, in that progesterone does *not* have an anti-proliferative effect.

Lack of detection of steroid receptors in fibroblasts suggests that stromal cells are not directly responsive to steroids. The menstrual cycle variation of proliferation in stroma suggests a role for local growth factors in control of proliferation in fibroblasts. Indeed, epithelial stromal interaction via autocrine mechanisms may be important in the co-ordination of proliferation in the two components of the breast.

ACKNOWLEDGEMENTS

The continued co-operation of the clinical staff at Longmore Hospital, Edinburgh and the technical assistance of Lorraine Allison and Lynda Ferrigan are gratefully acknowledged. The study was supported by the Imperial Cancer Research Fund.

REFERENCES

1. Anderson, T.J., Battersby, S., King, R.J.B., McPherson, K. and Going, J.J. (1989). Oral contraceptive use influences resting breast proliferation. *Hum. Pathol.*, **20**, 1139–44
2. Potten, C.S., Watson, R.J., Williams, G.T., Tickle, S., Roberts, S.A., Harris, M. and Howell, A. (1988). The effect of age and menstrual cycle upon proliferative activity of the normal human breast. *Br. J. Cancer*, **58**, 163–70
3. Battersby, S., Robertson, B.J., Anderson, T.J., King, R.J.B. and McPherson, K. (1991). Influence of menstrual cycle, parity and oral contraceptive use on steroid hormone receptors in normal breast. Submitted for publication

4. Lessey, B.A., Killam, A.P., Metzger, D.A., Haney, A.F., Greene, G.L. and McCarty, K.S. Jr. (1988). Immunohistochemical analysis of human uterine estrogen and progesterone receptors throughout the menstrual cycle. *J. Clin. Endocrinol. Metab.*, **67**, 334–40

SECTION 3

The high-risk patient and management

16

Pathological features as markers of breast cancer risk

R.A. Walker

INTRODUCTION

There is now a body of evidence which suggests that certain histopatho-
logically defined changes that can occur in women's breasts are markers
of increased risk of developing breast cancer. The evidence for this
comes from two main sources: the comparison of cancerous and non-
cancerous breasts, and the analysis and follow-up of patients who have
had biopsies for benign disease.

CANCEROUS AND NON-CANCEROUS BREASTS COMPARED

One of the first studies was that by Foote and Stewart[1] who reported
in 1945 that papillary hyperplasia with cytologic atypia was five times
more frequent in cancerous than non-cancerous breasts. They emphasized
that the terminal ducts within the breasts were the sites of hyperplasia
that were potentially precancerous. Bonser and colleagues[2] found that
cancerous breasts showed an increased incidence of epithelial hyperplasia
compared to autopsy controls, the frequency being up to 3.8 times
greater. Kern and Brooks[3] described a comparison of uninvolved areas
in mastectomies with specimens removed for fibrocystic changes, and
reported a greater incidence of atypical duct epithelial hyperplasia of a
borderline nature in the cancer-associated group.

A major study was that of Wellings and colleagues[4] who examined a wide variety of cancerous and non-cancerous breasts, including breasts contralateral to those with cancer, using a subgross sampling technique with histology. They identified a greater degree of atypical hyperplasia in cancerous breasts and those breasts contralateral to cancers than in non-cancerous breasts.

PROSPECTIVE ANALYSIS OF PATIENTS HAVING BENIGN DISEASE

There have been several prospective studies of women who have had biopsies for benign disease[5-9]. Page and colleagues[5] identified an increased risk of breast cancer if the biopsies contained ductal hyperplasia, papillary apocrine change and atypical lobular hyperplasia, the extent depending on the age of the patient. In a further study Dupont and Page[6] found that women having proliferative breast disease without atypia had a 1.9 times greater risk of developing breast cancer compared to women with non-proliferative lesions. The risk for atypical lesions was reported as 5.3 times that for women with no proliferative changes, and this increased to 11 times if there was a family history of breast cancer. A subsequent study[7] by the same authors considered that the risk of invasive breast carcinoma after atypical lobular or atypical ductal hyperplasia was 4–5 times that of the general population, with family history of breast cancer increasing the risk to 8 times for atypical lobular and 10 times for atypical ductal hyperplasia.

Hutchinson and co-workers[8] found an increased risk of breast cancer in women with fibrocystic change, characterized by epithelial hyperplasia, of up to 2.8 times. In a recent study by Tavissoli and Norris[9], the presence of atypia in epithelial hyperplasia was a significant factor in increasing the likelihood of developing a subsequent invasive carcinoma. However, this study commented on the vagueness of the criteria for separating atypical ductal hyperplasia from regular ductal hyperplasia and ductal carcinoma *in situ*.

PROBLEMS IN HISTOPATHOLOGICAL ASSESSMENT

The comments made in the above study emphasize the problems which are encountered when trying to subdivide precisely those changes in breast biopsies which indicate differing risks of development of breast cancer. The subjectivity of interpretation is well illustrated by the survey reported by Rosai[10], in which interobserver variability was assessed among a group of five experienced pathologists, and found to be unacceptably high. Interpretation of individual lesions ranged, in some cases, from regular hyperplasia through to carcinoma *in situ*.

OBJECTIVE EVALUATION OF AT-RISK LESIONS

There is a clear need for more objective criteria which will help to define the different at-risk lesions. The studies undertaken to attempt this have considered nuclear morphometry[11], DNA and proliferative analysis[12,13], tumour-associated antigen expression[14,15], and oncogene protein expression[16-18]. Nuclear area measurements can be of value for discriminating hyperplasia from carcinoma *in situ* but the position regarding atypia is less clear[11]. Some atypical hyperplasias have an abnormal DNA content[12], but DNA content cannot discriminate between atypical hyperplasia and carcinoma *in situ*, although mitotic counts are higher in the latter[13]. There are no clear-cut changes in the expression of tumour-associated markers[14,15]. While one group considered that there were certain differences in p21 *ras* protein expression between the different at-risk lesions[16], others have not[17]. C-erbB-2 protein has only been detected in ductal carcinoma *in situ* (40–60%, predominantly comedo type) and not in atypical lesions[18].

None of these studies have been performed on breast tissues from women who have subsequently gone on to develop breast cancer.

CONCLUSION

There are histopathological changes within breast biopsies which appear to indicate that a woman is at an increased risk of developing breast cancer. Assessment of the degree of risk is flawed by the subjectivity of the interpretation and currently, more specialized, objective approaches have failed to be of help.

REFERENCES

1. Foote, F.W. and Stewart, F.W. (1945). Comparative studies of cancerous versus non-cancerous breasts. *Ann. Surg.*, **119**, 573–90
2. Bonser, G.M., Dossett, J.A. and Tull, J.W. (1961). *Human and Experimental Breast Cancer*. (London: Pitman Medical)
3. Kern, W.H. and Brookes, R.N. (1969). Atypical epithelial hyperplasia associated with breast cancer and fibrocystic disease. *Cancer*, **24**, 668–75
4. Wellings, S.R., Jenson, H.M. and Marcum, R.G. (1975). An atlas of subgross pathology of the human breast with special reference to possible precancerous lesions. *J. Natl. Cancer Inst.*, **155**, 231–73
5. Page, D.L., Zwang, R.V., Rogers, L.W., Williams, L.T., Walker, W.E. and Hartmann, W.H. (1978). Relation between component parts of fibrocystic disease complex and breast cancer. *J. Natl. Cancer Inst.*, **61**, 1055–63
6. Dupont, W.D. and Page, D.L. (1985). Risk factors for breast cancer in women with proliferative breast disease. *N. Engl. J. Med.*, **312**, 146–51
7. Page, D.L., Dupont, W.D., Rogers, L.W. and Rados, M.S. (1985). Atypical hyperplasia lesions of the female breast. *Cancer*, **55**, 2698–708
8. Hutchinson, W.B., Thomas, D.B., Hamlin, W.B., Roth, G.J., Peterson, A.V. and Williams, B. (1980). Risk of breast cancer in women with benign breast disease. *J. Natl. Cancer Inst.*, **65**, 13–20
9. Tavassoli, F.A. and Norris, H.J. (1990). A comparison of the results of long-term follow-up for atypical intraductal hyperplasia and intraductal hyperplasia of the breast. *Cancer*, **65**, 518–29
10. Rosai, J. (1991). Borderline epithelial lesions of the breast. *Am. J. Surg. Pathol.*, **15**, 209–21
11. Bhattaccharjee, D.K., Harris, M. and Faragher, E.B. (1985). Nuclear morphometry of epitheliosis and intraduct carcinoma of the breast. *Histopathology*, **9**, 511–16
12. Crissman, J.D., Visscher, D.W. and Kubus, J. (1990). Image cytophotometric DNA analysis of atypical hyperplasias and intraductal carcinomas of the breast. *Arch. Pathol. Lab. Med.*, **114**, 1249–53
13. de Potter, C.R., Praet, M.M., Slavin, R.E., Verbeck, P. and Roels, J.H. (1987). Feulgen DNA content and mitotic activity in proliferative breast disease. A comparison with ductal carcinoma in situ. *Histopathology*, **11**, 1307–19
14. Ohuchi, N., Page, D.L., Merino, M.J., Viglione, M.J., Kufe, D.W. and Schlom, J. (1987). Expression of tumour-associated antigen (DF3) in atypical hyperplasias and *in situ* carcinomas of the human breast. *J. Natl. Cancer Inst.*, **79**, 109–17

15. Tavassoli, F.A., Jones, M.W., Majeste, R.M., Gratthawer, G.L. and O'Leary, T.J. (1990). Immunohistochemical staining with monoclonal Ab B72.3 in benign and malignant breast disease. *Am. J. Surg. Pathol.*, **14**, 128–33

16. Thor, A., Ohuchi, N., Horan Hand, P., Callahan, R., Weeks, M.O., Theillet, C., Lidereau, R., Escot, C., Page, D.L., Vilas, V. and Schlom, J. (1986). Ras gene alterations and enhanced levels of ras p21 expression in a spectrum of benign and malignant human mammary tissues. *Lab. Invest.*, **55**, 603–15

17. Ghosh, A.K., Moore, M. and Harris, M. (1986). Immunohistochemical detection of *ras* oncogene p21 product in benign and malignant mammary tissues in man. *J. Clin. Pathol.*, **39**, 428–34

18. Gusterson, B.A., Machin, L.G., Gullick, W.J., Gibbs, N.M., Powles, T.J., Elliott, C., Ashley, S., Monaghan, P. and Harrison, S. (1988). C-*erb*B-2 expression in benign and malignant breast disease. *Br. J. Cancer*, **58**, 453–7

17

Bioactive prolactin as a breast cancer risk marker

P.R. Maddox

PROBLEMS WITH PROLACTIN MEASUREMENT

The role of prolactin in rodent mammary carcinogenesis is now well established but the role of prolactin in human breast cancer remains controversial. This stems from two main points. Firstly, a failure of many studies to date to take into account the chronobiology of prolactin, leading to a lack of standardization of sampling methods. Secondly, almost all of these studies have used a radioimmunoassay to measure prolactin in human serum. The radioimmunoassay gives a highly sensitive and specific physical measurement of the amount of polypeptide hormone present in human serum. However, a bioassay measures the biological activity of the hormone, which after all is what we are really interested in. The problem with bioassays for prolactin measurement in the past has been a lack of accuracy and precision, for example the notorious pigeon crop-sac assay.

PROLACTIN BIOASSAY

This all changed however, when Tanaka and co-workers in Canada[1] developed a new sensitive and specific bioassay for lactogens in 1981. This bioassay utilizes the Nb2 node lymphoma cell (derived from a lymph node of an oestrogenized rat that developed a lymphoma) which

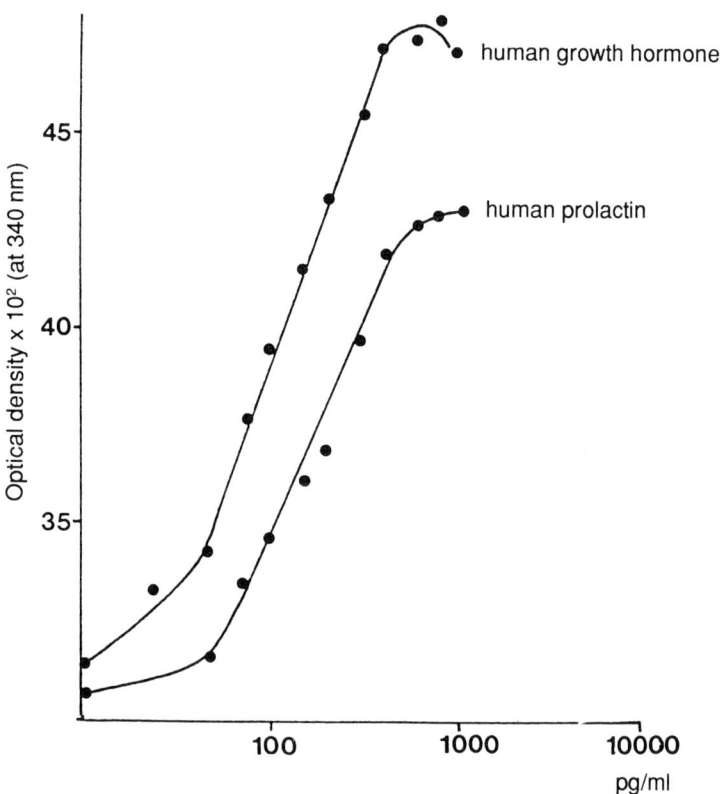

Figure 1 Standard curves for the growth of Nb2 cells measured by optical density in the presence of human prolactin and human growth hormone

will only divide the presence of lactogens. Growth of the cells over 3 days incubation correlates well with prolactin concentration in the culture medium leading to a standard curve. The three prime lactogens in human serum are prolactin, growth hormone and human placental lactogen, the latter being absent in the non-pregnant state. Specificity for prolactin is therefore afforded by the addition of an excess of anti-human growth hormone to the culture medium. Addition of varying concentrations of lactogen to the culture medium correlates well with cell mass after 3 days growth for both prolactin and growth hormone (Figure 1). The original method has been modified by scaling it down ten times to use microtest plates, and measuring cell mass by optical density using a spectrophotometer instead of the laborious Coulter counter technique to produce a more convenient and reliable microbio-assay, with no loss of sensitivity and an acceptable intra-assay and inter-assay variation for a biological assay[2].

PROLACTIN IN BREAST CANCER

A previously described increase in prolactin bioactivity in patients with breast cancer[3,4] stimulated an interest in looking further at women with familial breast cancer risk.

We know that 20–30% of women with breast cancer will have a family history of the disease, which remains the strongest clinical risk factor (apart from previous contralateral disease) with a ratio of up to 4 : 1[5]. From the work of Dupont and Page[6], we know that this risk will increase to the order of 7 : 1 if there has been a previous biopsy of atypical epithelial hyperplasia. Recently, Love and Rose[7] have described an increased prolactin bioactivity, up to 15 times that measured by radioimmunoassay, in a small number of women with a strong family history (at least two direct family members with the disease), but these findings have not been reproduced by other workers[8] and therefore I wished to examine this further.

METHODS

The aims of this work were therefore to measure basal and dynamic bioactive prolactin levels in women with a strong family history at risk of developing breast cancer, and also to assess the discriminating potential of prolactin bioactivity for breast cancer risk. Eighteen women with increased familial breast cancer risk, each having at least one direct family member with the disease were examined. The mean age was 45 years, two-thirds being premenopausal, and these women were compared to an age-matched control group. Both basal and dynamic prolactin levels were taken in the luteal phase, between 09.00 and 12.00, to standardize measurement. Bioactive prolactin levels were measured by the microbioassay (BA) described above, and radioimmunoassay (RIA) prolactin by the automated twin-site immunoradiometricassay.

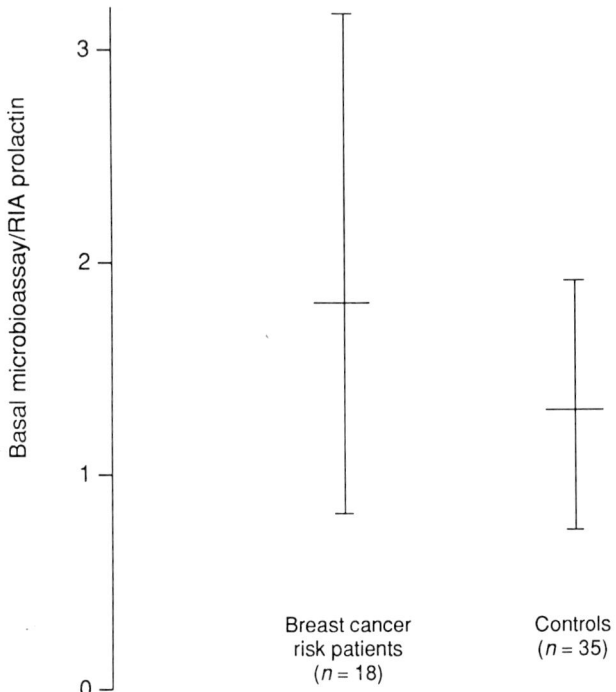

Figure 2   Basal BA/RIA prolactin ratios for breast cancer risk subjects and controls, showing means and ranges. (Mann–Whitney *U* test, breast cancer risk patients vs. controls, *p* < 0.02)

Both assays were standardized to International Reference Preparation 83/562.

RESULTS

Basal samples revealed no obvious difference in RIA levels between breast cancer risk patients and controls but microbioassay prolactin levels in the breast cancer risk group were found to be elevated over controls. This was best expressed as the ratio of BA to RIA (to give an index of prolactin bioactivity) which revealed a statistically significant difference between the breast cancer risk group and controls for the total group (1.8 vs. 1.4, *p* < 0.02). However, there was a great deal of overlap (Figure 2) and therefore it is unlikely to be a useful discriminator for breast cancer risk. The correlation of basal BA prolactin levels with age revealed a loss of the normal negative correlation for breast cancer risk women with a marked positive correlation for the premenopausal subgroup, which had a Pearson correlation coefficient of $r = +0.74$, indicating an increased prolactin bioactivity with age.

Dynamic levels were carried out using the stimulatory thyrotrophin releasing hormone (TRH) test. It was found that there were conventional rises after TRH stimulation for both BA and RIA prolactin levels in the control group. In the breast cancer risk group however, there was an exaggerated response for BA prolactin levels which was significantly greater than in controls, and was best demonstrated in the BA:RIA prolactin ratio for peak levels (Figure 3). It would therefore seem that the increased dynamic prolactin bioactivity may more closely reflect the prolactin status of women at breast cancer risk.

Investigation of the discriminatory potential of absolute and relative levels of prolactin bioactivity for basal and dynamic levels (expressed as the peak TRH response) revealed that the dynamic BA:RIA prolactin ratio was the most sensitive, showing elevated levels in 50% of the total and 75% of the premenopausal subgroup of breast cancer risk patients. Whether this increased prolactin bioactivity will prove to be a causal link with breast cancer and subsequently be translated into disease remains to be seen, and these patients are currently under close surveillance in the Cardiff Breast Clinic.

CONCLUSIONS

This work has demonstrated that basal and dynamic BA prolactin levels were significantly elevated in women with familial breast cancer risk, with a loss of the normal negative correlation of basal bioactive prolactin with age. Peak thyrotrophin releasing hormone BA:RIA prolactin ratio was the best discriminator of breast cancer risk from controls, and this measure of prolactin bioactivity may prove to be a useful biomarker of breast cancer risk, but further work is needed to substantiate this finding. This increased biological activity of prolactin in women with familial breast cancer risk also indicates that variant non-immunogenic forms of prolactin (or enhancing serum factors) must be present in the

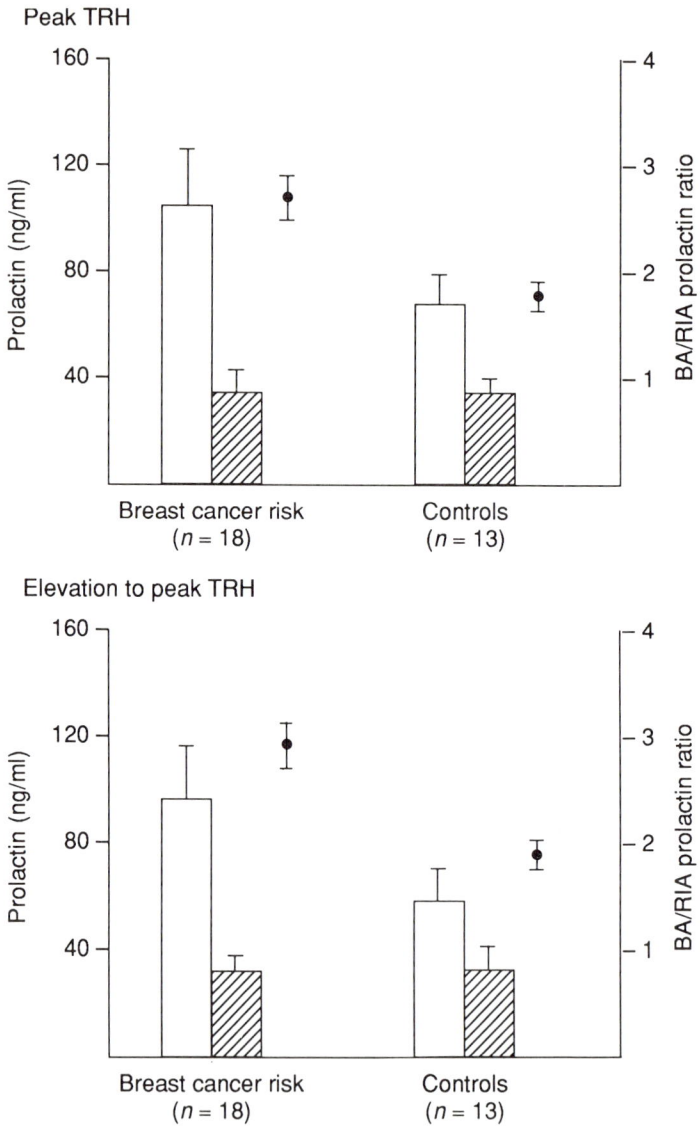

Figure 3 Peak TRH prolactin levels (mean ± SEM) by bioassay (BA) (empty bars) and radioimmunoassay (RIA) (hatched bars) for total breast cancer risk group and controls. The BA/RIA prolactin ratios are shown by ●. Mann–Whitney U test, breast cancer risk vs. control: BA, $p =$ NS; RIA, $p =$ NS; BA/RIA, $p < 0.002$

sera of women with breast cancer risk, as we have previously described for patients with breast cancer[3,4].

REFERENCES

1. Tanaka, T., Shiu, R.P.C., Gout, P.W. *et al.* (1980). A new sensitive and specific bioassay for lactogenic hormones: measurement of prolactin and growth hormone in human serum. *J. Clin. Endocrinol. Metab.*, **51**, 1058–63
2. Maddox, P.R., Jones, D.L. and Mansel, R.E. (1989). A new microbioassay for the measurement of lactogenic hormones in human serum. *Horm. Res.*, **32**, 218–23
3. Maddox, P.R., Jones, D.L. and Mansel, R.E. (1988). A new microbioassay for prolactin measurement; elevation of the bioactive/radioimmunoassayable prolactin ratio in breast cancer. *Br. J. Surg.*, **75**, 601
4. Maddox, P.R., Jones, D.L. and Mansel, R.E. (1988). Bioactive prolactin in breast cancer. In Ioannidou-Mouzaka, L., Philippakis, M. and Angelakis, P. (eds.) *Mastology '88*, pp. 403–6. (Amsterdam: Elsevier Science)
5. Stoll, B.A. (1991). Quantifying the risk of breast cancer. *Eur. J. Surg. Oncol.*, **17**, 36–41
6. Dupont, W.D. and Page, D.L. (1989). Relationship to previous breast disease. In Stoll, B.A. (ed.) *Women at High Risk to Breast Cancer*, p. 47. (Dordrecht: Kluwer)
7. Love, R.R. and Rose, D.P. (1985). Elevated bioactive prolactin in women at risk for familial breast cancer. *Eur. J. Cancer Clin. Oncol.*, **21**, 1553–4
8. Anderson, E., Morten, H., Wang, D.Y. *et al.* (1989). Serum bioactive lactogenic hormone levels in women with familial breast cancer and their relatives. *Eur. J. Cancer Clin. Oncol.*, **25**, 1719–25

18

Latent effects in the interpretation of any association between oral contraceptives and breast cancer

K. McPherson

INTRODUCTION

The epidemiological results of investigations into any possible association between oral contraceptives (OCs) and breast cancer appear quite conflicting. Several well-conducted cohort studies suggest rather strongly that long-term OC use is not associated with any change in breast cancer incidence, with the possible exception of one study. Most case–control studies also indicate overall no particular grounds for concern, with some important exceptions. Vital statistics in the form of mortality rates or registration rates also can be taken to be reassuring, but again with one or two non-trivial exceptions.

The epidemiological evidence will be reviewed in this paper to some extent, although the main purpose is to discuss the implication of particular kinds of biological mechanism on the interpretation of the epidemiology. Epidemiological studies tend to be interpreted by assuming that the investigated possible causative mechanisms of disease have immediate effect. Thus it is assumed, often implicitly, that if OC use does have an effect on breast cancer such an effect manifests itself immediately after use, for sufficient duration. Any study, therefore, which indicates no association is taken, perhaps quite mistakenly, to mean there is no causative effect, whereas a more precise interpretation might be that there is no effect which manifests itself immediately or in the short term. Clearly, such evidence does not exclude a delayed effect, unless much relevant exposure happened a long time before the diagnoses of breast cancer.

For many chronic diseases like breast cancer, time delays between exposure to risk factors and diagnosis of disease can sometimes be as long as several decades, and hence new and rapidly changing exposures like the use of OCs may therefore be coupled with great uncertainty in the interpretation of their epidemiological relationships. In the example to be discussed here, the implications are important, because firstly OC use is common, but also breast cancer is the most frequent female cancer among Western communities. Hence, since a biological association is *a priori* highly plausible, the potential for a large ultimate attributable risk is extremely important.

In the investigation of these matters it is obvious that such uncertainties cannot be finally resolved until sufficient time has elapsed to enable definitive study of any (delayed) relationship. However, in the interim, several investigations can throw important light on the scientific and policy questions. These concern the modelling of plausible effects with a view to understanding what effect they could have on contemporary epidemiology, so that current studies can be interpreted more completely. Since, until sufficient time has elapsed, the main problem will be a paucity of relevant data, it is also as well to understand the power against these hypotheses, and the precision of current studies.

EVIDENCE REGARDING AN ASSOCIATION BETWEEN ORAL CONTRACEPTIVES AND BREAST CANCER

There have been many epidemiological studies of the relationship between oral contraceptive use and subsequent breast cancer risk. Most show no (immediate) association and this evidence has been taken to be reassuring. Breast cancer is one of the commonest cancers among females in the developed world and it clearly has a hormonal aetiology, and hence any observed epidemiological association with OC use would be both plausible and extremely important.

Broadly, cohort studies, which were mostly begun in the 1960s soon after OCs became available, have shown little cause for concern. Long-term OC use has not been shown to be associated with any change in breast cancer risk[1]. Only one cohort study[2] has reported an elevated risk from use at any time of OCs, but only for breast cancer at a young age. A useful review of this association by Prentice and Thomas[3] using meta-analysis shows a relative risk of (essentially) unity for OC use and breast cancer. This appears to be as true among long-term pill users and for use 10–20 years before diagnosis.

The overall summary of case–control studies included in the overview of Prentice and Thomas also suggested no extra risk associated with OC use for many years and many years before diagnosis, but a relative risk of around 1.3 for prolonged use before first term pregnancy. Additionally, Schlesselman[4] has described an increasing risk with increasing duration of exposure before first term pregnancy when averaging over all published studies.

Several case–control studies have been published which do appear to show an association between OC use at a young age (described as early OC use) and breast cancer[5–9]. These studies are by no means unanimous, of course, and there are several recent studies which seem to show no association[10–12]. OC use before first term pregnancy or use at a young age is clearly an important subgroup in this context.

The most recent results of the National Case–Control study in the UK, of breast cancer and oral contraceptives among women under the age of 36, estimated a relative risk of up to 1.7 for 8 years of total OC use. Since it is recent it combines the most up-to-date information on the association with a high proportion of very young OC users. It is important to recognize that there is a necessary association between exposure to OCs at a young age and being currently young (see below).

The association of OCs and breast cancer could be of major public health significance if such risks as these found among under-35-year-olds are not confined to this age. There have been large changes in the extent, timing and type of OC use by different cohorts and any association of early OC use is therefore difficult to study reliably. This is particularly so since OC use at particular times in a woman's life may have quite a different effect on breast cancer risk.

Some have argued persuasively that the positive associations in the literature may be attributable to survey biases inherent in observational case–control study methodology[13]. It is always difficult finally to exclude such explanations from particular observational studies, and hence they remain plausible causes of some or all of the discrepancies. However it also remains possible that the largest negative study[11] has been incorrectly reported as being negative[14,15].

The fact that recent worrying studies are all case–control studies may be a reflection of the fact that cohort studies, which were mostly started in the late 1960s, concentrate on pill use at that time among women who were users then. Paradoxically, as we shall see, this may make them less relevant than contemporary case–control studies.

THE POSSIBILITY OF LATENT EFFECT

The notion that a latent effect could be important has received some attention[16,17]. Such a latent interval could include an induction period, during which time a single cancer cell is evolving, and a preclinical period, the time between the first cancer cell and the diagnosis of cancer. If we examine epidemiological studies of breast cancer, several features emerge as being possibly relevant to the interpretation of the association with OCs. A relatively young age at menarche is found to have a higher risk[18], also late age at first full-term pregnancy is a risk factor[19]. Breast cancer is uncommon until the mid-forties and hence age at menarche or first birth, if primary risk factors, must operate with a 'latent' interval of 30 years and more in some cases.

Moreover, diethylstilboestrol, a drug introduced in the 1940s and 1950s to prevent miscarriage, has been shown to be associated with an increase in subsequent breast cancer incidence. One study[20], among 3000 exposed women and 3000 similar women who were not exposed to the drug, showed a relative risk of around 2 associated with exposure after 40 years of follow-up. After 20 years there was no divergence at all in the cumulative breast cancer incidence curves between exposed and unexposed women. Hence, any epidemiological investigation under-taken among these women during the first 20 years after exposure would have yielded estimated relative risks of around unity.

It is, therefore, entirely plausible that OCs could be associated with a delayed effect on breast cancer incidence. Hence, it remains plausible that contemporary epidemiology is yielding biased estimates of what may turn out to be the ultimate relative risk. These may be termed 'analytical' biases, as opposed to 'survey' biases referred to by Skegg[13], since if present they will arise from inadequate implied models of disease causation used in the analysis. Conventional statistical analysis implicitly assumes an immediate effect of exposure on risk.

If OCs affect early stage carcinogenesis when used at a young age, or act as co-initiators by affecting mitotic activity[21], then any alteration to observed risk might not happen for 20 or so years after accumulated use. Anderson and colleagues[22] have, for instance, demonstrated an increased rate of mitotic activity in the endothelial cells of the human breast among young women on OCs. This increase was confined to nulliparous women using the pill; hence a particular effect of OC use before first term pregnancy remains plausible for biological reasons.

USE PATTERNS OF ORAL CONTRACEPTIVES

OCs have not been used by women in similar ways during their existence since the early 1960s. At first, they were used largely by married women predominantly for family spacing. This is because at that time it was very difficult for unmarried women to be prescribed OCs. Gradually use patterns changed and later, during the 'swinging sixties', all sorts of cultural expectations and social behaviour dramatically changed. In the UK the early 1970s witnessed a sharp rise in the prevalence of OC use among teenagers: from around 15% of sexually active single women aged less than 20 in 1970, to 50% by 1975, to nearer 80% by 1980[23,24]. During this period the dose has decreased and the type of synthetic hormones used has also changed.

The important point is that widespread use of OCs by women in their teens (described here as early use) is a recent phenomenon, and it is more recent in some communities than in others. There is some evidence to suggest, for instance, that use of OCs by young women happened in the USA more recently than it had in the UK[17,25]. Very little can now be said about the effect of early OC use on breast cancer risk at age 40 or more, simply because the women who were commonly exposed are only now reaching this age.

We have previously derived the proportions of women in our studies undertaken at Oxford who had been exposed to OCs before first term pregnancy by calendar year of birth[26] (see Table 1).

Table 1 Early OC use (before first pregnancy) by birth cohort and duration (expressed as %)

Year of birth, 19–	OC use (years)			
	Never	< 4	4 +	n (= 100%)
< 29	99	1	0	621
30–34	97	3	0	641
35–39	94	5	1	268
40–44	86	12	2	496
45–49	59	29	12	154
50–54	43	43	14	48
55–59	5	63	32	147
60–64	4	58	39	426
65–69	17	81	2	447

THE CONSEQUENCES OF A LATENT EFFECT

A simulation model[16] can provide insights into how latency can confuse the interpretation of epidemiology. The extent of the effect is surprising and might be deemed to be unnecessarily alarmist, in the absence of hard evidence. However, while some studies show no evidence of a delayed effect[10–12], others do[6,9]. The apparent conflict between studies could be attributable to differences in the time at which early use became common among young women. If, for instance, such use is more recent in one country than in another then obviously, if there is a latent effect, the estimated relative risks may be correspondingly different.

Moreover, straightforward statistical arguments indicate that contemporary studies of this association will lack precision if the delay period is in fact around 20 years, because relevant exposure sufficiently long ago is currently rare. For instance in a recent study[26] only 1.4% of 351 controls aged less than 45 had used OCs before first term pregnancy more than 20 years before the diagnosis of their age-matched case. This is merely five women. Moreover, none of these five women had accumulated prolonged use by this time. Thus such apparent inconsistency in the epidemiology is itself consistent, therefore, with a latent effect.

In general, if there were an effect of the kind described above then the observed relative risk associated with a given exposure would be expected to firstly increase with increasing age of diagnosis and secondly

Table 2   Estimated relative risk of 4 + years early exposure among women of different ages, if the latent interval is Gaussian, with a mean of 15 years and standard deviation of 4 years, and if the ultimate relative risk is 3

Age (years)	Estimated relative risk
25–29	1.0
30–34	1.3
35–39	1.8
40–44	2.3

increase as recent exposure was omitted from the designation of exposure. Both of these characteristics are true of two of the latter studies.

If, for instance, one postulates that long-term use of OCs before first term pregnancy does increase the risk of breast cancer threefold ultimately, but the time between this effect and diagnosis is a mean of 15 years, with a standard deviation of 4 years, then studies which include women of different age groups, based on OC use patterns shown in Table 1, should yield estimates of relative risk as shown in Table 2.

Notice, therefore, that the recent estimate of a relative risk of 1.3 for 4 years of OC use among women under the age of 35 is wholly consistent with an ultimate risk of 3 and a delay of only 15 years on average, between accumulated exposure and diagnosis. This was almost exactly the risk observed in the UK National study among women in 1984–86.

Similarly, if the use patterns by birth cohort of Table 1 are a true reflection of actual use in the UK, then the estimated relative risk observed in case–control studies including only women of an age to have been exposed while young would progress as in Figure 1, if the latent interval is 15 years on average. The confidence limits in Figure 1 reflect the increasing age of breast cancer cases and controls, who may have been exposed while young, as time progresses. Thus increasing power will become available to test these hypotheses.

If these assumptions are at all realistic, then cancer incidence would only change gradually, as the cohort of women who had used OCs for prolonged periods while young reached an age when breast cancer becomes relatively common. Simulations again indicate the extent of

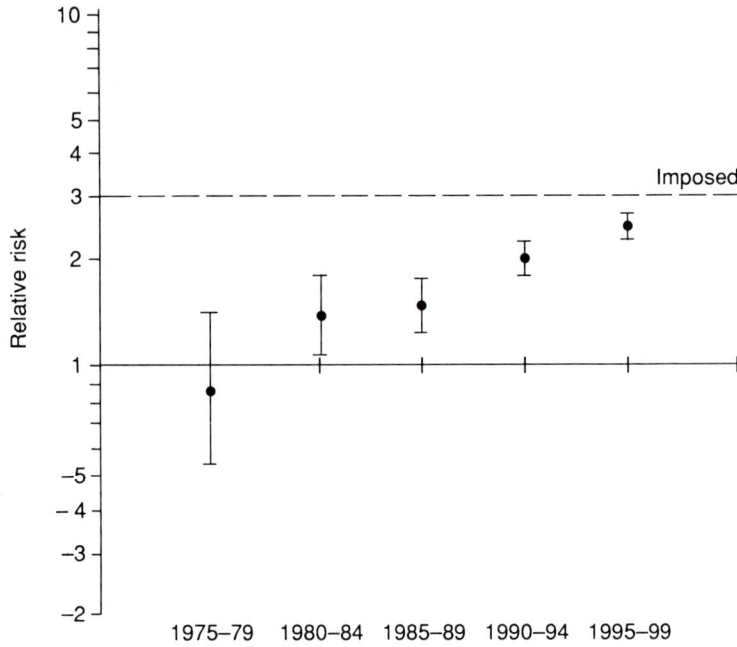

Figure 1 Estimated relative risk which would be observed in case–control studies, for women with 4 + years OC exposure before first term pregnancy vs. those with none. The 95% confidence limits are shown

this effect, making exactly the same assumptions as before. Because of early OC use patterns changing with time, the predicted changes among particular age groups might be shown in Table 3. It can be seen that only small changes in incidence would now be expected even if the relative risk is ultimately as high as 3. This is an unsatisfactory state of affairs because no detectable change in the incidence by 1985 might be expected, even if there is an important association. Currently, incidence figures for 1985 are published and are not inconsistent with Table 3. There are some increases among young women which are not consistent or worrying in themselves.

Fortunately, recent work from New Zealand contradicts these pessimistic arguments[27] but does not refute them, because the power against plausible risks remains very low. The massive Cancer and Steroid Hormone Study from the USA is often cited as strong evidence against

Table 3 Percentage increase in incidence of breast cancer among women of given age attributable to early OC use, if the ultimate relative risk associated with such use is 3, with an average delay of 15 years in England and Wales

Year	Age (years)			
	35–39	40–44	45–49	50–54
1981	0	0	0	0
1982	1	1	0	0
1983	2	1	0	0
1984	5	2	0	0
1985	7	4	1	0
1986	10	5	2	0
1987	13	6	3	1
1988	17	9	5	1
1989	21	12	7	2
1990	25	16	10	3
1995	41	36	31	14
2000	52	68	53	42

such an effect, but that was assuming it showed no effect of early OC use[11]. It is no longer clear that it does[14], although clarification is still awaited. Moreover the evidence does suggest that early OC use happened around 5 years later in the USA and, since the study was done in the early 1980s, an estimated relative risk of 1 must be interpreted like an estimated relative risk of 1 in 1975 in the UK. Both are wholly consistent with an ultimate relative risk of 3 combined with a latent period of 15 years.

Thus it is impossible to exclude a large effect of OCs on breast cancer incidence. Such an effect could ultimately change the lifetime risk of around one in 12 women to a lifetime risk of around one in four among those women who were long-term users of the pill early in their lives. Table 3 suggests that if these pessimistic assumptions are true, the incidence among all women aged 40–44 will increase by two-thirds by the end of this century. It is clear that ultimately the risk among older women, most of whom will have been exposed by the 2020s, might by then be doubled by common exposure to OCs while young.

Hopefully well before that time, the epidemiological evidence refuting such a prediction will be secure. It is not a foregone conclusion, however.

REFERENCES

1. Vessey, M.P., McPherson, K., Mackintosh, L. and Yeates, D. (1989). Oral contraceptives and breast cancer in a large cohort study. *Br. J. Cancer*, **59**, 613–18
2. Royal College of General Practitioners (1988). Breast cancer and the pill – A further report from the Royal College of General Practitioners' study. *Br. J. Cancer*, **58**, 675–80
3. Prentice, R.L. and Thomas, D. (1987). On the epidemiology of oral contraceptives and disease. *Adv. Cancer Res.*, **49**, 285–401
4. Schlesselman, J.J. (1989). Oral contraceptives in relation to cancer of the breast and reproductive tract. An epidemiological review. *Contraception*, **40**, 1
5. Pike, M.C., Krailo, M.D., Henderson, B. E., Cassagrande, J.J. and Hoel, D.G. (1983). Hormonal risk factors for breast cancer. *Nature (London)*, **303**, 767–70
6. McPherson, K., Vessey, M.P., Neil, A., Doll, R., Jones, L. and Roberts, M. (1987). Early oral contraceptive use and breast cancer: results of another case–control study. *Br. J. Cancer*, **56**, 653–60
7. Meirik, O., Lund, E., Adami, H.O., Bergstrom, R., Christofferson, T. and Bergsjo, P. (1986). Oral contraceptive use and breast cancer in young women. *Lancet*, **2**, 650–5
8. Miller, D.R., Rosenberg, L., Kaufman, D.W., Stolley, P., Warshaver, M. and Shapiro, S. (1989). Breast cancer before age 45 and oral contraceptive use: new findings. *Am. J. Epidemiol.*, **129**, 269–80
9. UK National Case–Control Study Group (1989). Oral contraceptive use and breast cancer in young women. *Lancet*, **1**, 973–82
10. Paul, C., Skegg, D.C.G., Spears, G.F.S. and Kaldor, J.M. (1986). Oral contraceptives and breast cancer: a national study. *Br. Med. J.*, **293**, 723–8
11. Stadel, B.V., Rubin, G.L., Webster, L., Schlesselman, J.J. and Wingo, P.A. (1985). Oral contraceptives and breast cancer in young women. *Lancet*, **2**, 970–4
12. Miller, D.R., Rosenberg, L., Kaufman, D.W., Schottenfeld, D., Stolley, P.D. and Shapiro, S. (1986). Breast cancer risk in relation to early oral contraceptive use. *Obstet. Gynecol.*, **68**, 863–8
13. Skegg, D.C.G. (1988). Potential for bias in case–control studies of oral contraceptives and breast cancer. *Am. J. Epidemiol.*, **127**, 205–12

14. Peto, J. (1989). Is the CASH study really negative? *Lancet,* **1**, 552
15. Stadel, B.V., Schlesselman, J.J. and Murray, P A. (1989). Oral contraceptives and breast cancer. *Lancet,* **1**, 1257–8
16. McPherson, K., Coope, P.A. and Vessey, M.P. (1986). Early oral contraceptive use and breast cancer – theoretical effects of latency. *Br. J. Epidemiol. Commun. Hlth,* **40**, 289–94
17. McPherson, K. (1988). Latent effect of oral contraceptives on breast cancer. *J. Am. Med. Assoc.,* **260**, 1240–1
18. Pike, M.C., Henderson, B.E., Krailo, M.D., Duke, A. and Roy, S. (1983). Breast cancer in young women and oral contraceptives: a possible modifying effect of formulation and age at use. *Lancet,* **2**, 926–31
19. McMahan, B., Cole, P. and Brown, J. (1973). Etiology of human breast cancer: a review. *J. Natl. Cancer Inst.,* **50**, 21–32
20. Greenberg, E.R., Barnes, A.B., Resseguie, L., Barratt, J.A., Burnside, S., Lanza, L.L., Neff, R.R., Stevens, M., Young, R.H. and Colton, T. (1984). Breast cancer in mothers given diethylstilbestrol in pregnancy. *N. Engl. J. Med.,* **311**, 1393–7
21. Buehring, G.C. (1988). Oral contraceptives and breast cancer: what has 20 years of research shown? *Biomed. Pharmacol.,* **42**, 525–30
22. Anderson, T.J., Battersby, S., King, R.J.B. and McPherson, K. (1989). Breast epithelial responses and steroid receptors during oral contraceptive use. *Hum. Pathol.,* **12**, 1137–43
23. Dunnell, K. (1976). *Family Formation,* Office of Population Censuses and Surveys. (London: Her Majesty's Stationery Office)
24. Bone, M. (1978). *The family planning services: changes and effects.* Office of Population Censuses and Surveys. (London: Her Majesty's Stationery Office)
25. Bachrach, C.A. (1984). Contraceptive practice among young American women 1973–1982. *Fam. Plann. Perspect.,* **16**, 253–9
26. McPherson, K. (1990). Summary and update of the Oxford-based studies. In Mann, R.D. (ed.) *Oral Contraceptives and Breast Cancer,* pp. 55–66. (Carnforth, UK: Parthenon Publishing)
27. Paul, C., Skegg, D.C.G. and Spears, G.F.S. (1990). Oral contraception and breast cancer in New Zealand. In Mann, R.D. (ed.) *Oral Contraceptives and Breast Cancer,* pp. 85–94. (Carnforth, UK: Parthenon Publishing)

19

Biochemical measurements in breast cyst fluid from patients developing subsequent carcinoma

W.R. Miller

INTRODUCTION

The composition of cyst fluids is distinctive[1] and cysts may be subdivided into major populations on the basis of, for example, the electrolyte profile of the fluid they contain[2]. Women with breast cysts seem to have a modestly increased risk of subsequent breast cancer[3,4] but it is still uncertain whether or not subgroups of cysts hold differing risk of breast cancer. The present study addresses this issue by identifying women with breast cysts who have subsequently presented with breast cancer. Cyst fluids from these women have been characterized for electrolyte type and levels of androgen conjugate and growth factors.

MATERIALS AND METHODS

Between 1981 and 1986, 1256 cysts were aspirated from 674 patients by needle aspiration. Fluids were centrifuged at $500 \times g$ for 5 min and the supernatant stored at $-20°C$ until assayed. Estimates of concentrations of sodium and potassium ions were performed by flame photometry on cyst fluids diluted in distilled water ($1:200$ v/v). Fluids having a sodium to potassium concentration ratio ($[Na^+]:[K^+]$) less than 4 were then classified as Group A, those with a ratio greater than 4 as Group B.

Androgen conjugates were measured by radioimmunoassay using an antibody described previously[5]. Epidermal growth factor (EGF) levels were measured by radioimmunoassay using a double antibody technique[6]. Levels of transforming growth factor-α (TGFα) were determined using a kit supplied by Peninsula Lab Inc, California. Statistical analyses were by Wilcoxon rank and chi-square tests as appropriate.

RESULTS

Follow-up by the Scottish Cancer Trials Office has identified 18 women who have gone on to develop breast cancer at least 1 year after cyst aspiration (cancers were diagnosed between 1 and 8 years later). The cyst fluid type of these patients is presented in Table 1. Although there was a tendency for Group A cysts to predominate, the proportion of Group A to Group B was not significantly different from that of the total study population.

In order to study further the comparative composition of cyst fluids derived from women subsequently presenting with breast cancer, these patients have been matched with women not developing breast cancer over the same study period, standardizing for the following criteria: date of cyst aspiration; multiplicity of cysts, both at presentation and during follow-up; and volume and electrolyte type of cyst fluid. Patients were also matched for age, menopausal status, parity and family history of breast cancer.

Matched cyst fluids have then been analysed for androgen conjugates, epidermal growth factor and TGFα. Results for androgen conjugates are shown in Figure 1. These show no significant difference in levels

Table 1 Electrolyte composition of cyst fluids in patients developing cancer (number in each group, followed by percentage)

	Cancers ($n = 18$)		Total study population ($n = 674$)	
	n	%	n	%
Group A	12	66	191	28
Mixture	3	17	286	42
Group B	3	17	197	29

$\chi^2 = 1.35$, NS

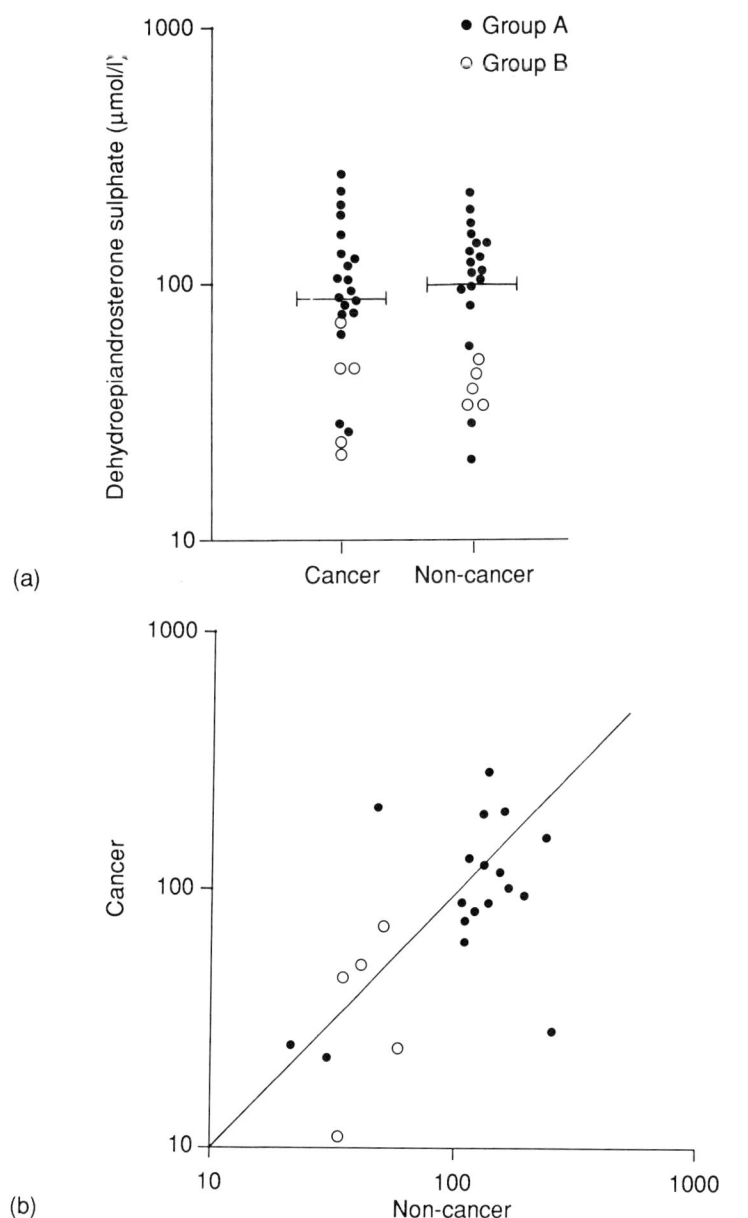

Figure I Levels of androgen conjugates in cyst fluids from women either subsequently developing breast cancer or not. (a) Group comparisons; (b) paired comparison

between cyst fluids from patients subsequently presenting with cancer and those not, although it is apparent that concentrations are markedly higher in Group A fluids as compared with Group B. Plotting the results as matched pairs of cancer and non-cancer individuals (right-hand panel) did not display any trend for values of androgen conjugates to be higher or lower in patients with subsequent cancer as compared with control women.

The corresponding data for EGF are shown in Figure 2. No significant difference in EGF levels was apparent between groups of women either presenting with subsequent cancer or not, although levels of EGF tended to be higher in Group A cysts. Individual pairing also failed to reveal a substantial trend towards either increased or decreased values in fluid from women having a subsequent breast cancer.

Results for TGFα are shown in Figure 3. Again no significant difference in TGFα levels was apparent between cyst fluids from women subsequently developing breast cancer and those not. This lack of discrimination is evident both in group and matched-pairs analysis.

DISCUSSION

These results show that the cyst type in patients subsequently developing breast cancer is not significantly different from the total population of cysts. However, a trend (which might have reached significance with greater numbers) was evident for women developing breast cancer to present with a greater proportion of Group A cysts. However, the picture is complicated by the problem of how to handle multiple cysts of mixed types. In so far as Group A cysts tend to predominate amongst them, and their clinical behaviour is similar to that of Group A cysts[7], it seems more logical to classify these with the Group A cysts. On this basis, the difference between patients subsequently presenting with cancer and the total population is further reduced. In the absence of an absolute correlation between Group A cyst fluids and presentation of breast cancer, the conclusion must be that electrolyte classification of cyst fluids alone cannot be used to predict appearance of cancer accurately.

Since other constituents of cyst fluids might be related to breast cancer risk, fluids have been analysed for hormones and growth factors which

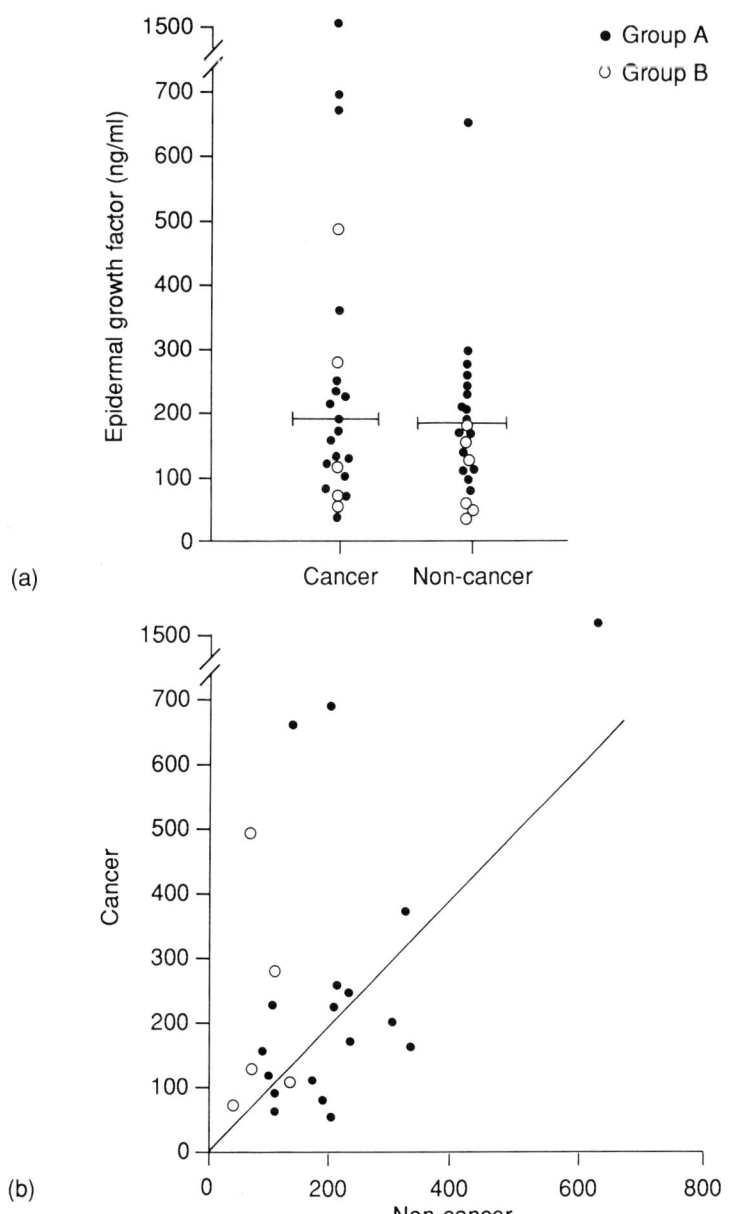

Figure 2 Levels of epidermal growth factor in cyst fluids from women either subsequently developing breast cancer or not. (a) Group comparisons; (b) paired comparison

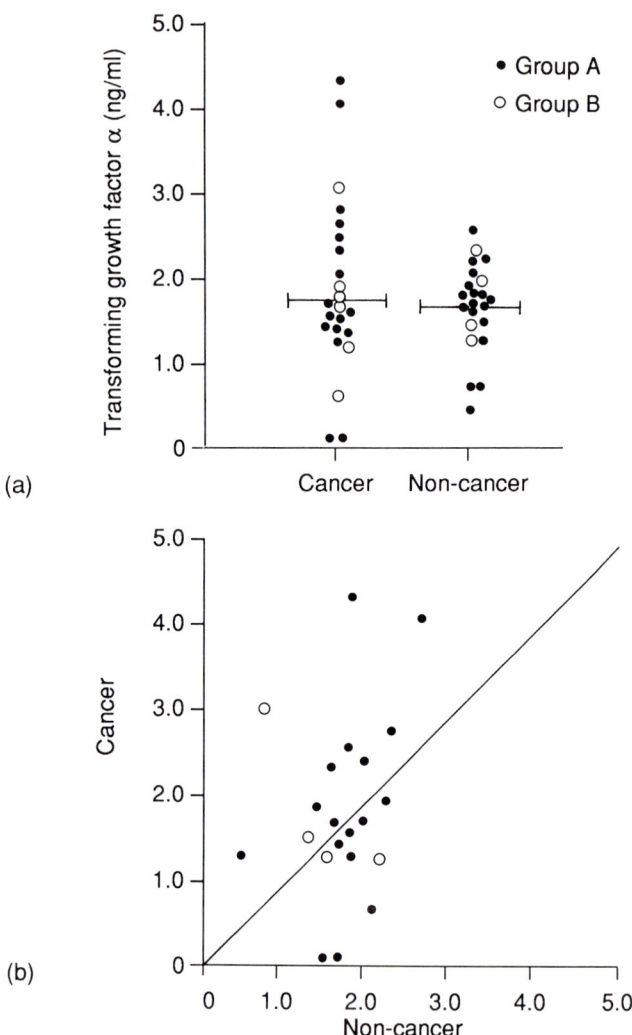

Figure 3 Levels of transforming growth factor-α in cyst fluids from women either subsequently developing breast cancer or not. (a) Group comparisons; (b) paired comparison

might have proliferative activity on breast epithelium. However, no significant difference in levels of androgen conjugates, epidermal growth factor and transforming growth factor-α were apparent between cyst fluids from patients developing breast cancer and those not. In some respects, these results are disappointing, but it should be emphasized that the development of breast cancer is multifactorial, and the measurement of factors which monitor proliferation but not the susceptibility or initiation of cancer are unlikely to be rewarding. Cyst fluids have been shown to contain mutagenic agents[8] and oncogene products[9] and their determination may yet prove to be more fruitful.

REFERENCES

1. Miller, W.R. (1990). Biochemistry of cyst fluids and its relevance. In Steroid formation, degradation and action in peripheral tissues. *Ann. N.Y. Acad. Sci.*, **595**, 459–63
2. Miller, W.R., Dixon, J.M., Scott, W.N. and Forrest, A.P.F. (1983). Classification of human breast cysts according to electrolytes and androgen conjugate composition. *Clin. Oncol.*, **9**, 277–32
3. Haagensen, C.D. (1986). *Diseases of the Breast*, 3rd edn., pp. 55–88. (Philadelphia: W.B. Saunders Co.)
4. Dupont, W.D. and Page, D.L. (1985). Risk factors for breast cancer in women with proliferative breast disease. *N. Engl. J. Med.*, **312**, 146–51
5. Miller, W.R., Humeniuk, V. and Kelly, R.W. (1980). Dehydroepiandrosterone sulphate in breast secretions. *J. Steroid Biochem.*, **13**, 149–51
6. Smith, K., Miller, W.R., Fennelly, J.A., Matthews, J.N.S., Scott, W.N. and Harris, A.L. (1989). Quantification of epidermal growth factor in human breast cyst fluids: correlation with dehydroepiandrosterone-sulphate and electrolyte concentrations. *Int. J. Cancer*, **44**, 229–32
7. Dixon, J.M., Scott, W.N. and Miller, W.R. (1985). Natural history of cyst disease: importance of cyst type. *Br. J. Surg.*, **71**, 190–2
8. Scott, W.N. and Miller, W.R. (1991). Mutagens in human breast cyst fluids. *J. Cancer Clin. Oncol.*, **117**, 254–8
9. Papamichalis, G., Francia, K., Karachalioy, F.E., Anastasuades, O.T. and Spandidos, D.A. (1988). Expression of the c-*myc* oncoprotein in human metaplastic epithelial cells of fibrocystic disease. *J. Anticancer Res.*, **8**, 1217–22

20

The Royal Marsden Hospital prevention trial

M.C. Nicolson and T.J. Powles

THE RATIONALE

Breast cancer is currently responsible for 20% of female cancer deaths. Its incidence is increasing and cure rates are not improving. An alternative approach to control of the disease is to prevent its development. Adjuvant tamoxifen can reduce the incidence of breast cancer in the contralateral breast by 45%[1]. To investigate whether tamoxifen can prevent breast cancer in healthy women at high risk of developing the disease, a double-blind randomized trial was initiated at the Royal Marsden Hospital in 1986.

THE TRIAL

Eligible women, usually aged over 40 years, with a family history of breast cancer, not at risk of pregnancy and able to give informed consent are randomized to receive either tamoxifen (20 mg daily) or placebo. In this intervention study involving healthy people, it is imperative to monitor drug safety carefully. A potential 'antioestrogen' given to healthy women could cause thromboembolic disease, osteoporosis and ischaemic heart disease. The effect on the uterus and ovaries must also be assessed because of a possible increase in endometrial carcinoma[2].

At 6-monthly intervals, the women in our study are assessed for compliance and acute toxicity, and have a clinical breast examination. Annually they have mammography, pelvic ultrasound scan, measurement of bone mineral density, measurement of blood coagulation factors (fibrinogen and antithrombin-3) and lipid assessment.

RESULTS

Compliance is excellent, monitored at 80% for tamoxifen and placebo at 3 years after randomization. This is partly due to the low acute toxicity. Of the toxicities reported, the two significantly more common in the tamoxifen-treated group are hot flushes (34% tamoxifen vs. 18% placebo) and vaginal discharge (9% tamoxifen vs. < 1% placebo). That tamoxifen's effect is selectively oestrogenic is confirmed by lack of significant alteration in fibrinogen levels or in the fibrinogen/antithrombin-3 ratio at any time up to 3 years after randomization. There is no difference in the age-corrected bone mineral content between the two groups. Plasma cholesterol is significantly reduced in the tamoxifen-treated group, and is maintained at 15% lower than pre-randomization levels in both pre- and postmenopausal women. The effect is most marked in those women who have a high initial cholesterol level. Further lipid analysis confirms a significant reduction in the low density lipoprotein cholesterol component and in the apolipoprotein-b, thus suggesting a possible protective effect of tamoxifen against ischaemic heart disease. The cardioprotective high density lipoprotein cholesterol is increased in tamoxifen-treated women, but not significantly so.

CONCLUSION

With 850 healthy but high-risk women already randomized to receive either tamoxifen or placebo, it is obviously possible to accrue good numbers into the study. This highly motivated and altruistic group of women have maintained 80% drug compliance up to 3 years after randomization. No untoward side-effects have been documented, and tamoxifen may exert a cardioprotective effect as evidenced by the significant, maintained reduction in serum cholesterol.

The main question – whether breast cancer can be prevented by tamoxifen given to high-risk women – remains unanswered at this early stage of the study. Ethical clearance has now been gained to recruit 1500 women at the Royal Marsden Hospital. We would expect to see a difference in breast cancer development between the tamoxifen- and placebo-treated group in the next 5 years, but the results may be apparent earlier because of extension of the study to national level, when 15 000 women will be included.

REFERENCES

1. Cusick, J. and Baum, M. (1985). *Lancet*, **2**, 282
2. Fornander, T., Rutquist, L.E. and Cedermark, B. (1989). *Lancet*, **1**, 117

SECTION 4

How I do it

21

How to measure psychological morbidity in women with benign breast disease

S.J. Leinster

INTRODUCTION

Psychological factors may play a part in the presentation of women with benign breast disease, in particular, cyclical mastalgia. This possibility can only be excluded by measurement of psychological parameters.

SELECTION OF PARAMETERS FOR MEASUREMENT

There is no single entity which equates to 'psychological well-being'. The selection of the appropriate psychological test depends on the identification of the psychological dimensions which are likely to be abnormal. It is important, therefore, that there be an *a priori* hypothesis which predicts the parameters which should be measured.

There are now accepted, well-documented psychological concepts which can be reliably measured. It is, in general, better to use these dimensions rather than attempting to develop new, apparently specific, measures. If it is felt necessary to introduce a new measure, it should be used alongside an existing measure so that comparison can be made with other groups which have been well characterized.

Attempts have been made to produce a global 'quality of life' score, particularly for cancer patients[1]. The concept is attractive but has proved less than satisfactory in practice. In order to produce a global figure, weighting has to be given to the different components of the score[2]. No agreement exists as to the magnitude of the weightings. It is better to measure and report individual dimensions, thus allowing the readers to make any value judgements.

SELECTION OF INSTRUMENTS FOR MEASUREMENT

Selection of appropriate controls

In any study of psychological parameters in benign breast disease, it is essential that appropriate controls be selected. In studies on the prevalence of cyclical mastalgia in Merseyside[3] and Cardiff[4], it was found that 60–70% of women on direct questioning admitted to experiencing cyclical mastalgia. Only 3.4% of the Merseyside women had ever sought treatment for their symptoms.

In looking for psychological factors leading to a presentation with breast disease, there should be a control group of women suffering from the symptom but not presenting for treatment, in addition to a totally asymptomatic group. It is, of course, important that the controls be matched as far as possible with the symptomatic group with respect to other variables, such as age and parity, which might have an effect on the symptoms.

Selection of tests

There are a number of issues which must be addressed with respect to the test instruments chosen[5].

Tests can be classified as nomothetic or idiographic. Nomothetic tests have been tested against reference populations and have norm values for the variables being tested.

Idiographic tests do not have any external reference but are useful for comparing changes in a patient with time. A common example of the idiographic test is the visual analogue scale for pain commonly used in trials of the treatment of cyclical mastalgia. This allows comparison of the patient's perception of symptoms before and after treatment. Mean scores before and after treatment for a group of patients can legitimately be compared, but it is not possible to compare the score of one patient with that of another patient in a meaningful way.

In general, nomothetic tests are to be preferred as they allow a better comparison of the symptomatic group with the general population.

Tests should be valid, reliable and responsive. The testing of validity is a formal matter and construct validity is, perhaps, the most useful measure of validity. There is a tendency to accept 'face' validity when new tests are introduced – 'it looks as if it tests X', but this is unsatisfactory as confounding variables may be affecting the test and factors other than the obvious may be giving rise to the test scores. The only value of face validity is that subjects are more likely to complete the test if it appears to fulfil its ostensible purpose.

Similarly, reliability should be formally tested and not assumed. Responsiveness is the ability of the test to detect small but real changes in a given subject with time. It is closely tied to reliability. Any difference in score between the test administered on different occasions should be due to changes in the subject and not to random error in the instrument.

Validity and reliability rely on correlation statistics for their derivation. A newer approach to the same problem ('does the test measure what we think it does?') is the concept of generalizability. This depends on analysis of variance for its derivation and may be a more accurate assessment of a test[6].

These considerations mean that it is better to select a standard instrument for a given study than to attempt to derive a new instrument, as the verification of the new instrument is a lengthy and complicated procedure. Any new instrument which is produced to cover some particular facet of the patients should be used in conjunction with well-tried instruments so that comparison can be made between studies.

Selection of an appropriate protocol

Cyclical mastalgia is a cyclical phenomenon, so the tests should be administered in the follicular and luteal phases of the cycle. The administration of the tests could have some placebo effect on the symptoms and the pretreatment testing should take place on more than one occasion to exclude this effect.

EXAMPLE OF APPROACH USED

Our consideration of the available data led us to hypothesize that women with cyclical mastalgia who presented for treatment would be more anxious than normal symptomless women or those with cyclical mastalgia who do not present for treatment. We also postulated that the patients would display cyclical mood change.

The basic instrument we chose to examine these hypotheses was the Hospital Anxiety and Depression scale[7]. This scale has been designed for use with patients with organic disease and excludes somatic symptoms from the assessment of anxiety and depression. Some other scales may give spurious results because symptoms arising from the organic condition may be scored as arising as a result of psychological morbidity. The scale has been well validated and is both reliable and responsive.

A deficiency of the Hospital Anxiety and Depression scale is that it tests the mental state at the time of administration. Since a patient with mastalgia may be anxious or depressed because of the persistence of her symptoms, another test was necessary to examine the patient's underlying tendency to anxiety. For this purpose we used the Spielberger State/Trait Anxiety questionnaire[8].

Using these measures, we have shown that the women who present for treatment are more anxious than either of the control groups. This is true both for state (current) and trait (underlying) scores. They also have a marked mood swing with the cycle having higher scores for anxiety and depression in the luteal phase of the cycle. These mood changes can be eliminated by hormonal treatment.

CONCLUSION

Further studies are necessary to establish the role of psychological factors in the aetiology of cyclical mastalgia. These studies should use accepted, properly evaluated instruments and should report the individual components of scores rather than attempting to derive a global quality of life score.

REFERENCES

1. Maguire, P. and Selby, P. (1989). Assessing quality of life in cancer patients. *Br. J. Cancer*, **60**, 437–40

Measurement of psychological morbidity

2. Olschewski, M. and Schumacher, M. (1990). Statistical analysis of quality of life data. *Stat. Med.*, **9**, 749–63
3. Leinster, S.J., Whitehouse, G.H. and Walsh, P.V. (1987). Cyclical mastalgia: clinical and mammographic observations in a screened population. *Br. J. Surg.*, **74**, 220–2
4. Maddox, P. and Mansel, R.E. (1988). The treatment of cyclical mastalgia. *Breast News*, **2**, 4-6
5. Owens, R.G. (1984). Psychological assessment. In McGuffin, P., Shanks, M.F. and Hodgson, R.J. (eds.) *The Scientific Principles of Psychopathology*, pp. 505–21. (London, Orlando and New York: Academic Press)
6. McReynolds, P. (1975). *Advances in Psychological Assessment*, Vol. **3**, pp. 60–70. (San Francisco: Jossey Bass)
7. Zigmond, A.S. and Snaith, R.P. (1983). The Hospital Anxiety and Depression scale. *Acta Psychiatr. Scand.*, **67**, 361–70
8. Spielberger, C.D. (1983). *State-Trait Anxiety Inventory.* (Palo Alto, CA: Consulting Psychologists Inc.)

22

Fine needle aspiration cytology

J.M. Dixon

INTRODUCTION

Fine needle aspiration cytology is now the investigation of choice to diagnose solid breast lumps[1-4]. It has considerable advantages over other diagnostic techniques in that it is less traumatic, it can be performed at the patient's first attendance and gives highly accurate results[4,5]. British studies have reported failure to obtain satisfactory samples in 3–48% of all cancers[6-9]. The major factor which has been reported to influence cytology results is the experience of the operator[4,5,10,11]. For this reason, all fine needle aspirates in our unit are performed by designated, experienced aspirators.

METHOD

I use a 10 ml syringe and a 21-gauge (green) needle for fine needle aspiration of breast lumps. There is no reason why a smaller syringe cannot be used, but studies have suggested that a 21-gauge needle produces optimal results[12]. I do not use an aspiration gun as I think this reduces the sensitivity of the procedure.

The lesion to be aspirated is identified, firstly by examination with the right hand, and is then fixed between the index and middle fingers of the left hand. I rarely, if ever, fix the lesion between finger and thumb. The method of fixation I use has the advantage of moving the palpable lesion over a rib, with the fingers pressing down into the surrounding intercostal spaces, and it therefore reduces the risk of a pneumothorax. To date, despite performing over 3500 fine needle aspirates, I have not seen a pneumothorax in a patient I have aspirated.

The skin overlying the lesion is wiped with an alcohol-soaked swab and the needle on the syringe is then introduced through the skin over the lesion and advanced until an abnormal area is identified with the tip of the needle. The plunger is pulled back to between 3 and 5 ml and the needle passed in and out of the lesion anywhere between 10 and 25 times, suction being maintained throughout. The number of passes through the lesion is determined by the amount of material aspirated. It is difficult to obtain a satisfactory aspirate from some lesions and these require more passes.

At the end of aspiration, the plunger is allowed to return to the zero mark before the needle is withdrawn. The material in the barrel of the needle and the syringe is then expressed onto a series of microscope slides and spread. Care is taken not to place too much material on each slide. Half the slides are air dried and the other two are spray fixed in alcohol. Slides are then stained by Giemsa and Papanicolaou techniques, respectively.

For very small or very superficial breast masses, either a 23-gauge (blue) or 25-gauge (orange) needle has advantages. I find these lesions easier to identify with a smaller needle. If the clinical abnormality is small and cannot be fixed between two fingers, it is possible to fix these very small lesions either under the left index or left middle finger, introducing the needle just beyond the tip of the finger.

Some lesions are very vascular and large amounts of blood are aspirated almost immediately on introducing the needle. In these patients, the needle is withdrawn and a further attempt at aspiration performed in a different direction, usually using a smaller (23-gauge) needle. Where a second aspirate is being performed after an initial bloody aspirate, flushing the syringe and needle with heparin prior to repeating the aspiration does stop clotting and may be useful. I have not found the routine use of heparin of any value in increasing diagnostic yield. It is important, if there is blood in the aspirate, that the slides are prepared as quickly as possible so that clotting of the specimen does not occur.

Breast fine needle aspirates should be reported by experienced breast cytopathologists, as this reduces the rate of false positives while not reducing the sensitivity of the technique.

RESULTS

Table 1 shows the accuracy of fine needle aspiration cytology in the diagnoses of 516 breast carcinomas performed by multiple or single aspirators. It is clear from publications from the majority of other breast units in the United Kingdom that aspirates in these centres are still being performed by a large number of aspirators, and this probably explains why the results from centres which use designated aspirators have consistently been the best obtained in this country[1,5,13].

BENIGN DISEASE

Fine needle aspiration cytology can be used to confirm a benign diagnosis and thus avoid biopsy[13]. Table 2 shows the results obtained from a series of benign lesions. A number of benign lesions, particularly those benign lesions in elderly women, are poorly cellular and, despite an adequate aspirate being performed, they do not contain any epithelial cells and are therefore reported as acellular. I am happy to accept an acellular aspirate, in the absence of any clinical or mammographic suspicion, as confirming the diagnosis of benign disease. Where there is any clinical or mammographic suspicion, then an acellular aspirate should be repeated

Table 1 Accuracy of fine needle aspiration cytology in the diagnosis of 516 breast carcinomas when performed by multiple or single aspirators

Cytological diagnosis	Multiple aspirators		Single aspirators	
Malignant	114	} 59%	262	} 99%
Suspicion of malignancy	26		14	
Benign	33		1	
Acellular	63		3	

Table 2 Fine needle aspiration in 372 benign lesions

Cytological diagnosis	n	%	
Malignant	0	0	
Suspicious	16	4.3	
Benign	275	73.9	} 95.7%
Acellular	81	21.8	

Table 3 Immediate reporting of patients referred from a screening clinic with 152 palpable lesions

Management	n
Fine needle aspiration only (no biopsy)	40
Biopsies	
total	112
malignant	81
benign	31
benign/malignant	0.38

as it may be unrepresentative and, therefore, unsatisfactory. It is clear from our experience that the majority of acellular aspirates are not 'inadequate', a term used by some pathologists. Where a fine needle aspirate confirms that a lesion is benign, then I am happy to manage such a lesion by observation only and would only excise it if this was the patient's wish. Contrary to what many surgeons believe, the majority of patients with benign lumps are happy to keep them[13].

FINE NEEDLE ASPIRATION WITH IMMEDIATE REPORTING

Fine needle aspiration cytology with immediate reporting has been used in Edinburgh for some time. Immediate reporting does not seem to reduce the accuracy of this technique[6,12]. Table 3 shows how fine needle aspiration cytology influences the management of patients referred with palpable lesions from breast screening. Using cytology, the benign-to-malignant ratio is considerably below that suggested as adequate in the Forrest report[14].

CONCLUSION

Fine needle aspiration cytology performed by an experienced aspirator is the most accurate available technique to diagnose the nature of solid breast lumps, other than surgical excision. Management of breast lumps in our unit is based largely on the results of fine needle aspiration cytology.

REFERENCES

1. Zajdela, A., Ghossein, N.A., Pilleron, J.P. and Ennuyer, A. (1975). The value of aspiration cytology in the diagnosis of breast cancer: experience of the Foundation Curie. *Cancer,* **35,** 499–506
2. Schöndorf, H. (1978). *Aspiration Cytology of The Breast.* (Philadelphia: W.B. Saunders)
3. Zajicek, J. (1974). *Monographs in Clinical Cytology. I. Aspiration Biopsy cytology.* (Basel: Karger)
4. Dixon, J.M., Anderson, T.J., Lamb, J., Nixon, S.J. and Forrest, A.P.M. (1984). Fine needle aspiration cytology in relationship to clinical examination and mammography in the diagnosis of a solid breast mass. *Br. J. Surg.,* **71,** 593–6
5. Dixon, J.M., Lamb, J. and Anderson, T.J. (1983). Fine needle aspiration of the breast: importance of the aspirator. *Lancet,* **2,** 564
6. Duguid, H.L.D., Wood, R.A.B. and Irving, A.D. (1979). Needle aspiration of the breast with immediate reporting of material. *Br. Med. J.,* **2,** 185–7
7. Davies, C.J., Elston, C.W., Cotton, R.E. and Blamey, R.W. (1977). Preoperative diagnosis in carcinoma of the breast. *Br. J. Surg.,* **64,** 326–8
8. Furnival, C.M., Hughes, H.E., Hocking, M.A., Reid, M.M.W. and Blumgart, L.H. (1975). Aspiration biopsy in breast cancer. *Lancet,* **2,** 446–8
9. Webb, A.J. (1970). The diagnostic cytology of breast carcinoma. *Br. J. Surg.,* **57,** 259–64
10. Ashley, S., Royle, G.T., Corder, A., Herbert, A., Guyer, P.B., Rubin, C.M. and Taylor, I. Clinical, radiological and cytological diagnosis of breast cancer in young women. *Br. J. Surg.,* **76,** 835–7
11. Barrows, G.M., Anderson, T.J., Lamb, J. and Dixon, J.M. (1986). Fine needle aspiration of breast cancer: relationship of clinical factors of cytology results in 689 primary malignancies. *Cancer,* **58,** 1493–8
12. Hartley, M.N., Tuffnell, D.J., Hutton, J.L., Palmer, M. and Al-Jafari, M.S. (1988). Fine needle aspiration cytology: an *in vivo* study of cell yield. *Br. J. Surg.,* **75,** 380–1
13. Dixon, J.M., Clarke, P.J., Crucioli, V., Dehn, T.C.B., Lee, E.C.G. and Greenall, M.J. (1987). Reduction in the biopsy rate in benign breast disease using fine needle aspiration cytology with immediate reporting. *Br. J. Surg.,* **74,** 1014–16
14. Forrest, P. (1986). *Breast Cancer Screening.* (London: Her Majesty's Stationery Office)

23

The management of nipple discharge

K. Horgan

INTRODUCTION

Nipple discharge is a common occurrence amongst the general female population but is a relatively uncommon reason for referral to a breast clinic[1]. It is almost invariably listed on health education leaflets as an important sign of breast cancer and therefore causes much unwarranted anxiety. Nipple discharge is an uncommon presentation for breast cancer and the vast majority of women with nipple discharge do not harbour a cancer.

MACROSCOPIC APPEARANCE

The management of nipple discharge is clinically based and depends on a clear description of its macroscopic appearance. Only discharges which are true, spontaneous, persistent and non-lactational are of importance[2]. True discharge comes directly from a duct or ducts and appears on the nipple. It excludes secretions due, for example, to skin eruptions or eczema, or those due to mammillary fistulae. The discharge should be spontaneous, arising with little provocation as most women can elicit some discharge with determined sustained manipulation.

The most important feature of a discharge is whether it is blood-related or not. Blood-related discharges can be serous (yellow), serosanguinous (pink) or bloody, and are associated in a minority of women with an underlying carcinoma. All other discharges, such as multicoloured, opalescent or milky types, are not associated with cancer. The only exception to this is the uncommon crystal clear, watery type. On first examination, therefore, the majority of women can be reassured that there is no worry with regard to malignancy.

BLOOD-RELATED DISCHARGES

Blood-related discharges are due to duct ectasia or hyperplastic epithelial lesions. Rough estimates attribute 50% to intraduct papillomata, 35% to duct ectasia and 15% to cancer. Exact figures for the duct ectasia component are not readily available as the pathological basis for the diagnosis is not always clear-cut. The risk of malignancy increases appreciably with age, especially in the postmenopausal group. Haagensen's[3] experience with serous and bloody discharge showed equivalent significance for both, whereas Leis[2] found a fivefold increased likelihood of cancer with blood-stained types. If there is a palpable breast mass then it takes precedence and is managed in the conventional manner. An associated nipple discharge does not increase the likelihood of a mass being malignant at any age. Devitt[4] found that a breast lump was almost invariably present when the nipple discharge was associated with a cancer while 13% of the cancers reported by Leis were without any palpable abnormality[2]. Both authors show that a very careful examination of the breast is warranted. This can be augmented by simultaneous ultrasound. Careful palpation of the breast will frequently reveal a particular area where pressure will maximize the discharge and therefore deserve special attention.

   Mammography is of use where it demonstrates abnormalities such as an impalpable carcinoma or calcification along the line of a duct indicative of ductal carcinoma *in situ*. A negative mammogram, especially in the older woman, does not obviate the need for a tissue diagnosis. Similarly, discharge cytology is useful when malignant cells are found but care must be taken in the interpretation of the results as approximately 2% false-positive rates occur. A negative finding should be ignored.

   We have not found ductography helpful. It may suggest an intraductal lesion but this is already suspected on clinical grounds; it does not alter the indications for surgery and it is an uncomfortable and disagreeable procedure for the patient.

Management of blood-related discharge

The management of blood-related nipple discharge is surgical. In a younger woman with discharge from a single duct and no other clinical or mammographic problem microdochectomy is sufficient. The duct is usually quite obvious, filled with bloody secretion and does not normally need any probe or dye localization. It should be followed peripherally if distended beyond the subareolar region, as very occasionally peripheral papillomata are found. The presence of intraduct papillomata is highly likely if the discharge from a single duct is relatively profuse. The papillomata are often multiple within a duct and are usually found immediately behind the nipple and areola. It is important to orientate the excised specimen for the pathologist. Frozen section histology has no role in the routine management of nipple discharge.

If the discharge is from multiple ducts or from a lady over 40 years old, total duct excision as described by Hadfield is the operation of choice[5]. This is also true for older women with a clear history of recent bloody nipple discharge which had ceased spontaneously. With careful attention to technical detail, Hadfield's procedure for nipple discharge in the absence of gross infection, or severe periductal mastitis, should result in very good cosmesis. It is especially important that the areola is not traumatized by forceps or excess diathermy coagulation and that the correct subvenous subcutaneous plane is found.

An uncommon but very distinct discharge is a crystal-clear watery type. It is the only non-blood related discharge with a cancer association though the malignant risk is disputed[2,3]. It must therefore be managed as for blood-related types.

NON-BLOOD-RELATED DISCHARGE

This group consists mainly of milky or opalescent multicoloured forms, though Leis[2] includes a third purulent type which is very uncommon in this context in our experience. Milky discharge or galactorrhoea is not related to any primary breast problem. It may be provoked by excessive expression or stimulation of the breast and the cessation of this practice together with explanation and reassurance of its self-limiting course is often sufficient for resolution. Galactorrhoea also occurs secondary to many drugs or prolactinomas. The detection rate of the latter has greatly improved with the advent of more sensitive measures of prolactin and computed tomographic scanning.

Opalescent discharges are most commonly yellow, white, green, brown or grey and may require treatment only if they cause embarrassment or distress for the patient. Major duct excision is the procedure of choice.

In summary, the overall management of nipple discharge is based on a recognition of its appearance, which should lead to a low incidence of surgery without omitting the removal of any neoplastic cause.

REFERENCES

1. Hughes, L.E., Mansel, R.E. and Webster, D.J.T. (1989). *Benign Disorders and Diseases of the Breast*, pp. 133–42. (London: Baillière Tindall)
2. Leis, H.P.L. Jr. (1989). Management of nipple discharge. *World J. Surg.*, **13**, 736–42
3. Haagensen, C.D. (1986). *Diseases of the Breast*, 4th edn. (Philadelphia: W.B. Saunders)
4. Devitt, J.E. (1985). Management of nipple discharge by clinical findings. *Am. J. Surg.*, **149**, 789–92
5. Hadfield, J. (1960). Excision of the major duct system for benign diseases of the breast. *Br. J. Surg.*, **48**, 472–7

24

Management of recurrent duct fistula

L.E. Hughes

INTRODUCTION

Sir Hedley Atkins first drew attention to duct fistula in Britain in his paper entitled '*Mammillary Fistula*' in 1955[1]. He reported 28 cases treated 'since the last war' and gave recognition to the precedence of the paper by Zuska, Crile and Ayres, who gave the first clear description in 1951[2]. These authors likened the condition to a fistula *in ano*, a similarity which appealed to Atkins, who recommended that it should be dealt with 'in a manner similar to that which has been so successful for fistula *in ano*'. Atkins reported no recurrence after adopting such an approach. Those who have experience of tertiary referral for both fistula *in ano* and mammary duct fistula may see more than an element of Freudian slip in the way Atkins draws a parallel between the excellent results from fistulotomy in both situations. Tertiary referrals show that the simple fistulotomy of Atkins or the fistulectomy of Patey[3] are both frequently followed by recurrence and there are many reasons for this. Perhaps the two main reasons are that fistulotomy is often used in inappropriate circumstances and is performed incorrectly where the circumstances are appropriate. Yet used appropriately and performed correctly, this simple fistulotomy of Atkins can give rise to very satisfying results.

CIRCUMSTANCES INDICATING SIMPLE FISTULOTOMY

Fistulotomy should be successful where the following criteria are met. A recurrent subareolar abscess discharges at the same single site, the nipple is everted or only moderately inverted and there is no inflammation peripheral to the fistula opening. In this type of case, a fine probe should be passed into the fistula opening and out through the affected duct on the surface of the nipple. The fistula is then laid open by a radial incision down onto the probe and the wound allowed to heal by granulation. Fistulectomy is a reasonable alternative to fistulotomy but this should be conservative, excising only sufficient scar tissue to reach normal tissue, thus minimizing damage to adjacent ducts and segments.

DEALING WITH RECURRENT FISTULA

In appropriate circumstances as outlined, and using this technique, a cure should be anticipated with mammary duct fistula. If recurrence occurs, a systematic assessment should be made of the possible causes (Table 1), and measures taken appropriate to the identified cause.

Inappropriate case selection

Mammary duct fistula is a disorder of a single duct and fistulectomy is not appropriate to cases with diffuse inflammation, either as a result of multiple duct involvement with periductal mastitis or extension of infection by surgery. The differentiation of a (single) duct fistula and more diffuse periductal mastitis is a complex matter[4]. The latter will not be cured by simple fistulotomy.

Table 1 Causes of recurrent infection following fistulotomy/fistulectomy for mammary duct fistula

---

Inappropriate case for fistulectomy
Residual central duct
Peripheral infection
Fibrotic subareolar abscess
Deep nipple inversion
Sebaceous cyst
Factitial disease

Residual central duct

Although on gentle manipulation a probe can usually be passed from the fistula right through the opening of the duct at the nipple, the terminal centimetre or so of the affected duct is found *in situ* surprisingly often when recurrent subareolar abscess and fistula develop after fistulotomy. The fistula should be cured by excising the persisting portion of duct.

Peripheral infection

Peripheral infection may occur in the same breast segment as the fistula. It is uncommon after simple fistulotomy but suggests more extensive duct ectasia with infection. The first approach should be a prolonged course of antibiotics for up to 4 weeks. If the infection recurs after this, it will require segmental excision of the abscess with the wound allowed to granulate.

Fibrotic subareolar abscess

This is seen more often after a Hadfield type procedure for periductal mastitis but may also occur after fistulectomy with primary wound closure rather than granulation. The dense fibrosis prevents proper drainage of the abscess with a persisting focus of infection. It requires a Hadfield type procedure allowing the wound to heal by granulation.

Deep nipple inversion

This is not cured by simple fistulotomy or fistulectomy and may act as a persisting source of infection, especially by staphylococci, into the subareolar space. It requires a Hadfield procedure and core nipple duct excision with nipple and areola preservation.

Sebaceous cyst

There are a number of large sebaceous glands in the nipple which may cause a recurrent abscess simulating a duct fistula. It is not cured by simple drainage and it does not communicate with a duct. It requires total excision of the cyst.

Factitial disease

This must be considered in unusual recurrent breast infections, especially in young to middle-aged women in medically-related professions. It is a diagnosis made on awareness and by exclusion. Sometimes total excision of the nipple or even mastectomy may be performed in an attempt to eradicate infection. It is important to avoid such unnecessary radical surgery for unusual infections and to consider self-mutilation as a possible cause.

REFERENCES

1. Atkins, H.J.B. (1955). Mammillary fistula. *Br. Med. J.*, **2**, 1473–4
2. Patey, D.H. and Thackray, A.C. (1958). Pathology and treatment of mammary duct fistula. *Lancet*, **2**, 871–3
3. Zuska, J.J., Crile, G.J. and Ayres, W.W. (1951). Fistulas of lactiferous ducts. *Am. J. Surg.*, **81**, 312–17
4. Hughes, L.E., Mansel, R.E. and Webster, D.J.T.W. (1989). *Benign Disorders and Diseases of The Breast*, p. 125. (London: Baillière Tindall)

25

Needle localization biopsy

U. Chetty

INTRODUCTION

The use of mammography as an aid to diagnosis or as a screening test presents the problem of mammographic abnormalities which are impalpable. There are three major categories of mammographic abnormalities associated with malignancy: microcalcification, parenchymal disturbances and mixed lesions. The assessment of the possibility of a malignancy associated with any particular feature is difficult and requires considerable training and expertise. In the management of these lesions, the whole process of the decision to operate, needle localization, surgery, confirmation of excision, and diagnosis requires close co-operation between the surgeon, radiologist and pathologist.

Fine needle aspiration cytology, performed under radiological or ultrasonographic guidance, is used increasingly to diagnose these lesions[1], though the problem of inadequate samples remains.

The aim of needle localization biopsy is either to diagnose the lesion or, in those cases proven on fine needle aspiration cytology to be a cancer, to treat the lesion. There are several methods available for placing a marker to guide the surgeon to the lesion[2]. If the mammographic lesion is visible on ultrasound, ultrasonic guidance can be used, which is the simplest method. However, areas of microcalcification may not be visible on ultrasound. Various devices are currently available to allow radiological guidance but the fundamental principle on which they are based remains the same. If a stereotactic pair of radiographs of an object are made, and given that the geometry remains known and constant, then the exact position of the small target area within the object can be located by calculation and allows the insertion of a fine wire marker.

Surgery is usually performed under general anaesthesia, though local anaesthesia can be used. It is important to be clear whether the localization biopsy is being done for a diagnostic purpose or as part of the treatment of a non-palpable cancer previously diagnosed by mammography or stereotactically obtained cytology. Surgery for the former is done as a biopsy taking a minimal margin around the lesion, while the latter is done as a wide local excision taking at least 1 cm of apparent normal breast tissue around the abnormality down to the deep fascia. Confirmation that the mammographic lesion has been excised must be obtained by specimen radiography and this must be compared to the original mammogram. The wound is closed only after it has been confirmed that the mammographic lesion has been fully excised.

The pathologist also has to be certain that he has examined the right part of the block of tissue and therefore, slicing of the specimen (about 4 mm thick) and X-raying of the slices is required.

For the efficient diagnosis of non-palpable lesions, a multidisciplinary team consisting of a radiologist, a pathologist and a surgeon is required to avoid, on the one hand, missing cancers and on the other, unnecessary biopsies. Continual monitoring of the quality of mammography and assessment is required. A regular review session by the team must be carried out, when individual cases are discussed and an audit made of malignant to benign ratio, interval cancer and missed cancer rates, accuracy of localization and complications.

REFERENCES

1. Freundlich, I.M., Hunter, T.B., Seeley, G.W., D'Orsi, C.J. and Sadowsky, N.L. (1989). Computer-assisted analysis of mammographic clustered calcifications. *Clin. Radiol.*, **40**, 295–8
2. Kirkpatrick, A.E. (1989). The radiological localisation of impalpable lesions. *Current Imaging*, **1**, 108–13

26

The problem of radial scars in breast screening

I.J. Monypenny, K. Lyons, N.S. Dallimore and K. Horgan

The introduction of the British national breast screening programme for all women between the ages of 50 and 64 has revealed an increased number of mammographic abnormalities with characteristics which are difficult to distinguish from those of malignancy. The presence of an area of asymmetric radial distortion must always be considered suspicious and warranting further evaluation; nevertheless a proportion of such lesions will subsequently be identified as benign radial scars.

The distinct histological entity of a central spindle of sclerosis and elastosis with varying degrees of epithelial proliferation and cystic change around the periphery has been recognized by a number of investigators at different times, leading to some confusion over nomenclature. This has included the terms radial scar[1,2], complex compound heteromorphic lesion[3], infiltrating epitheliosis[4] and indurative mastopathy[5]. However, general agreement has been reached on the use of the term 'radial scar' for smaller lesions up to 10 mm in size, and 'complex sclerosing lesion' for the larger ones[6]. Nevertheless, for the purpose of this paper, we have grouped all such lesions together loosely as radial scars.

The mammographic features of such lesions are of asymmetric distortion with strands radiating out from a central point. Usually, however, a mass lesion at the centre cannot be found and, moreover, there may be translucency, possibly due to fat entrapment. The lesions are often discoid in shape, thus being more apparent on one of the bi-planar views. They are frequently 10–20 mm in size, although much

213

larger radial scars can be found with no palpable abnormality. With ultrasound, radial scars are usually invisible or have non-specific appearances. Although such features raise the suspicion of a radial scar, discrimination between this and well-differentiated cancers such as tubular carcinomas is impossible without cytological or histological examination of tissue from the lesion. Stereotactic guidance is usually necessary to obtain fine needle aspiration cytology (FNAC) in the absence of any palpable or ultrasound abnormality, and may positively identify some of those lesions which are actually cancers. However, the reliability of negative cytology in excluding the presence of cancer is questionable because of the difficulties of obtaining adequate samples and of interpreting the aspirate from well-differentiated tumours.

Since the inception of the screening programme in south-east Wales in 1989, we have followed a policy of excising all screen-detected mammographic abnormalities which have been suggestive of radial scars according to the criteria described above. We have examined our results to date to determine the incidence of mammographic radial scars in the age-group of the screened population and to assess the wisdom of excising all such lesions.

In the first 24 months of the present round, 20 956 women were screened, of whom 967 (4.6%) were recalled for further assessment. An overall cancer detection rate of nine cancers per 1000 women screened has been obtained, with a benign/malignant biopsy ratio of 0.4. After full evaluation with detailed mammography, clinical examination, ultrasound and FNAC where indicated, 32 women were thought to have mammographic radial scars. All of these lesions have been excised, with wire localization if there was no palpable abnormality.

Histology showed that 28 of the mammographic lesions were true radial scars, giving an overall incidence of 1.34 per 1000 women screened. However, in three of these cases, *in situ* cancer was identified in the surrounding breast tissue as an incidental finding (two cases of ductal and one of lobular carcinoma *in situ*). Four of the mammographic 'radial scars' were identified histologically as cancers (two tubular carcinomas, one Grade 1 invasive ductal and one invasive lobular carcinoma). In total, therefore, histology revealed that 22% (7/32) of the mammographic 'radial scars' contained cancer changes.

These data show that mammographic areas of radial distortion of the type discussed are a moderately common finding in the prevalent round of a breast screening programme. Differentiation from cancers can be difficult on mammographic, clinical and ultrasound criteria. Although FNAC may identify a proportion of the cancers in this group, the considerable expertise needed to carry out the stereotactic FNAC which is required in the majority of such lesions may limit its value to specialist centres. Furthermore, since cells are obtained from the mammographic lesion, it is possible to miss the *in situ* cancer which we have found associated with 10% of our series of true radial scars. Although the accuracy of FNAC in this context requires further evaluation, at present we must recommend that all radial scars should be excised for definitive histological examination unless unequivocally malignant FNAC has been obtained.

REFERENCES

1. Hamperl, H. (1975). Strahlige Narben und obliterierende mastopathie. Beitrage zur pathologischen histologie der mamma. XI. *Virchows Arch. (A)*, **369**, 55–68
2. Linell, F., Ljungberg, O. and Andersson, I. (1980). Breast carcinoma. Aspects of early stages, progression and related problems. *Acta Pathol. Microbiol. Scand. (A)*, **272** (Suppl.), 1–233
3. Wellings, S.R., Jensen, H.M. and Marcus, R.G. (1975). An atlas of subgross pathology of the human breast with special reference to possible precancerous lesions. *J. Natl. Cancer Inst.*, **55**, 231–73
4. Azzopardi, J.G. (1979). *Problems in Breast Pathology*, pp. 174–87. (Philadelphia: Saunders)
5. Rickert, R.R., Kalisher, L. and Hutter, R.V.P. (1981). Indurative mastopathy: a benign sclerosing lesion of the breast with elastosis which may simulate carcinoma. *Cancer*, **47**, 561–71
6. Andersen, J.A., Carter, D. and Linell, F. (1986). A symposium on sclerosing duct lesions of the breast. *Pathol. Annu.*, **21**, 145–79

27

Benign lesions radiologically mimicking malignancy – anecdotes from a Forrest Breast Screening Unit

P.B. Guyer

INTRODUCTION

The aim of the Breast Screening Units set up on the recommendation of the Forrest report[1] is the early detection of breast cancer. The system will inevitably also detect a number of benign abnormalities and with some of these it may be necessary to go to biopsy to establish the precise diagnosis. This will adversely affect the benign : malignant ratio, which is one of the parameters which is used in the quality assurance of the breast screening process, and which Forrest recommended should be less than 3 : 1. The general experience across the country has been that this ratio is 0.5–1.5 : 1.0; but this is still not as good as is achieved in the more experienced Swedish breast screening programme. This, and the anecdotes described here, are two reasons why perhaps an improvement in the benign : malignant ratio in the UK can be anticipated. The abnormalities concerned are mainly hyalanized fibroadenomata, complex sclerosing lesions (radial scars), and atypical microcalcifications. Intracystic carcinoma and phyllodes tumours may also be difficult to diagnose accurately.

SMALL MASSES OBSERVED ON MAMMOGRAMS

Small, well-defined masses up to 1 cm in diameter are commonly observed on screen mammograms. Our initial reaction was to recall all these lesions for assessment, on the basis that up to 2% of them might be malignant (for example, mucinous carcinoma), but they were so numerous that a policy was adopted that, unless there were uncertain radiological features about these lesions, they were left without excision. A worrying feature which was detected in 15 of these during the first 2 years of screening (approximately 25 000 patients) was the finding of increased attenuation on ultrasound deep to some nodules, mimicking carcinoma. The surgical excision of these 15 lesions resulted in a diagnosis of hyalanized fibroadenoma[2]. Six of the nodules showed a clear echo-bright zone between the nodule and the deep attenuating shadow (Figure 1) suggesting that the lesion might be benign, and nodules showing this zone are now being observed rather than excised. Given these suspicious imaging features and the fact that a negative fine needle aspiration cytology may represent faulty sampling, biopsy then has to be considered on the imaging features alone. Fine needle aspiration cytology was, in fact, attempted on five of these lesions, producing benign cells in three, and an inadequate sample in two.

PHYLLODES TUMOURS

These appear similar to fibroadenomas, except that on X-ray about 25% will show rather coarser calcifications than those which are characteristic of fibroadenomas. With ultrasound, about one-third of phyllodes tumours will show internal fluid clefts or spaces[3], and fine needle aspiration may produce benign cells. If none of these features are identified, these tumours remain as usually well-defined, solid masses which are frequently quite large, and which will have to be considered for excision.

An occasional occurrence has been the detection of ductal *in situ* carcinoma within a fibroadenoma. In a screening programme, both these conditions are to be expected, and the reason for excision of these lesions has been atypical microcalcifications within a well-defined mass. Our view has been that the concurrence is coincidental (Figure 2) and we do not regard this as evidence to support any suggestion that a fibroadenoma may occasionally turn into a malignant lesion, although one of the carcinomas showed some invasion.

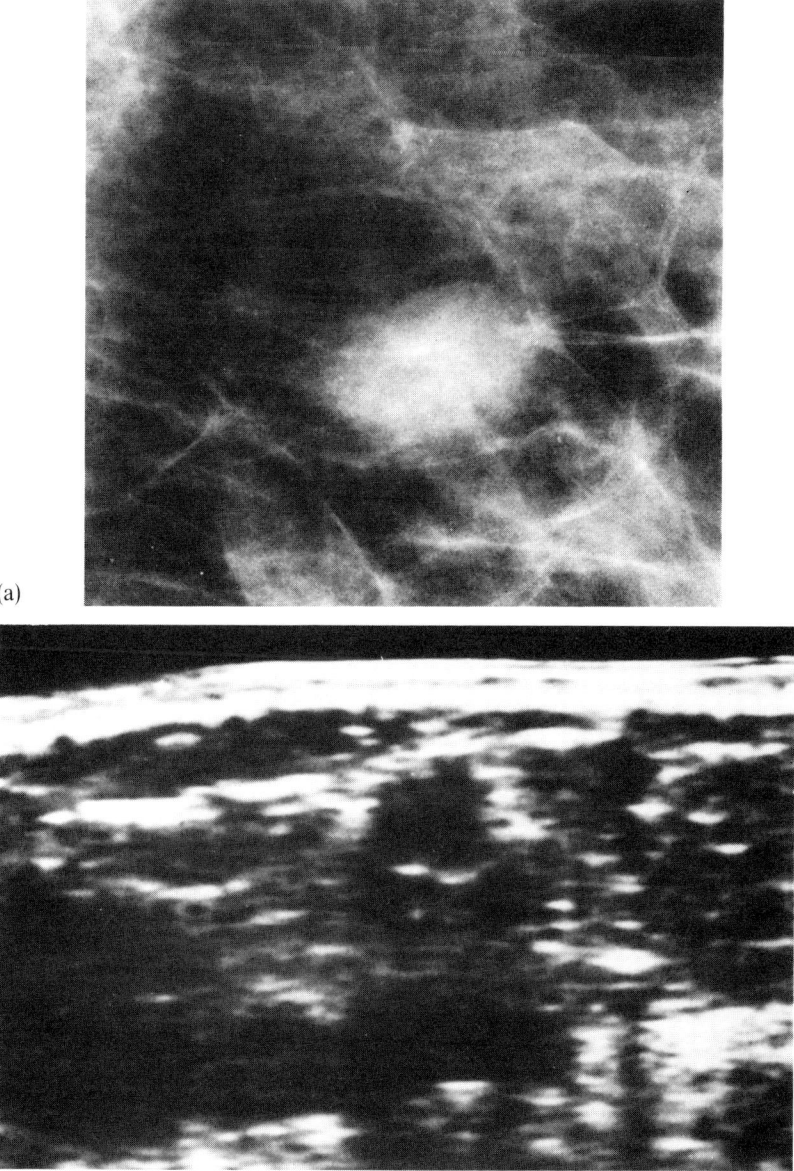

(a)

(b)

Figure 1 Hyalanized fibroadenoma: (a) the X-ray mammogram showing a nodule which lacks border definition in places; patient recalled for assessment; (b) ultrasound shows an echo-poor nodule separated from retro-tumourous attenuation by a narrow echo-bright zone. Biopsy showed an hyalanized fibroadenoma

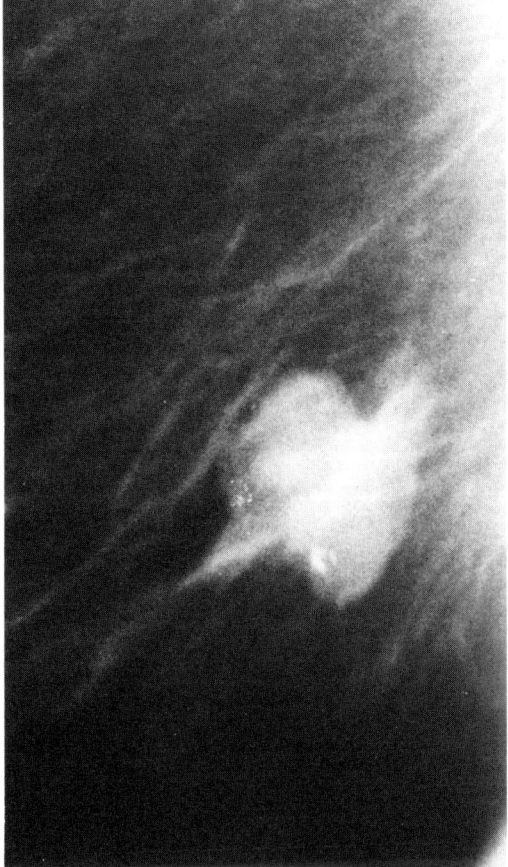

Figure 2 Carcinoma within a fibroadenoma: the nodule is well-defined superiorly and inferiorly, but in the midplane apparently striated. There is a mixture of amorphous calcification superiorly and punctate microcalcification posteriorly. Biopsy showed an intraduct carcinoma within a fibroadenoma

INTRACYSTIC MASSES

In our experience intracystic masses have always proved to be benign, even though the occurrence of intracystic carcinoma is well recognized. These have been detected during the assessment of a circumscribed solitary mass on the X-ray mammogram, and typically are well shown by ultrasound (Figure 3). Excision is necessary for certainty of diagnosis.

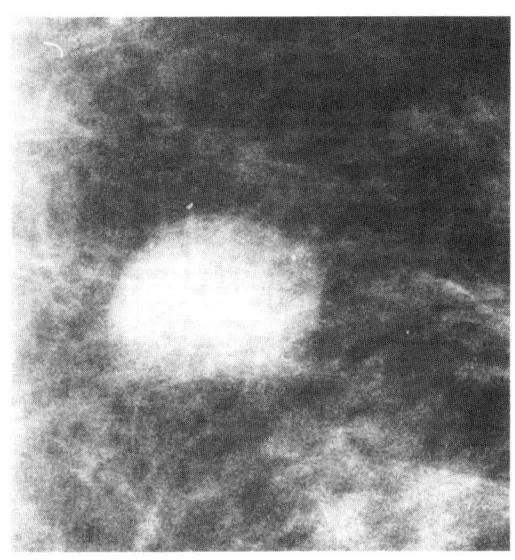

(a)

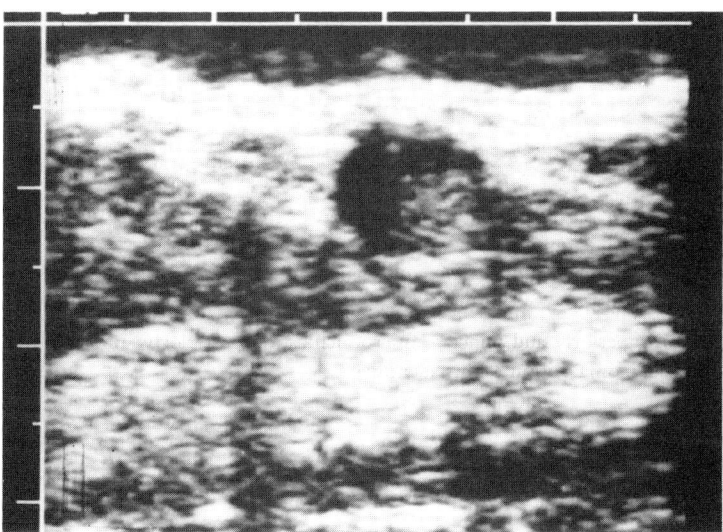

(b)

Figure 3 Intracystic papilloma: (a) solitary well-defined nodule deep to the areola; (b) ultrasound shows intracystic nodule. Biopsy showed an intracystic papilloma

RADIAL SCARS

Radial scars (complex sclerosing lesions) are a frequent finding histologically[4], but are much less commonly detected radiologically (Figure 4). Their nature is debated[5]. Monypenny and colleagues (Chapter 26) record a frequency of 1.34 per 1000 screen mammograms, but these appear to include examples of stromal deformity which radiologically our unit would conclude were probably benign. We always assess such stromal abnormalities, but use ultrasound as a parameter for decisions on surgery: if ultrasound is negative a watching policy is employed, whereas if ultrasound shows attenuating shadow, in association with the stromal deformity, then surgery is recommended on the basis of possible malignancy. Indeed, some of these radial scars are radiologically indistinguishable from carcinoma, and, even if fine needle aspiration cytology is negative, our policy has become to excise all such suspicious abnormalities (Figure 4)[6]; carcinoma has been described in association with them (see Chapter 26).

MICROCALCIFICATIONS

Microcalcifications may present great diagnostic problems, and have locally contributed significantly to the number of benign excisions. They can safely be left when layering of calcium is visible ('teacups'), or when there is a typical morular formation[7], but local stromal fibrosis, as in sclerosing adenosis (Figure 5), may alter the morphology of the microcalcifications, making differentiation from malignant lesions impossible[8,9]. In this case biopsy is essential for diagnosis.

DUCT ECTASIA

This has been a surprise histological diagnosis in some masses detected in our unit, in which there was preoperative suspicion of malignancy (Figure 6). These masses shown on X-ray mammography have been of variable size and shape, with some poor definition of outline, and even

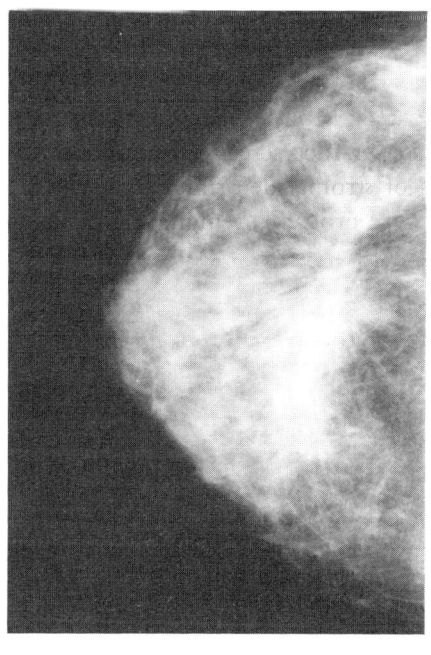

(a)

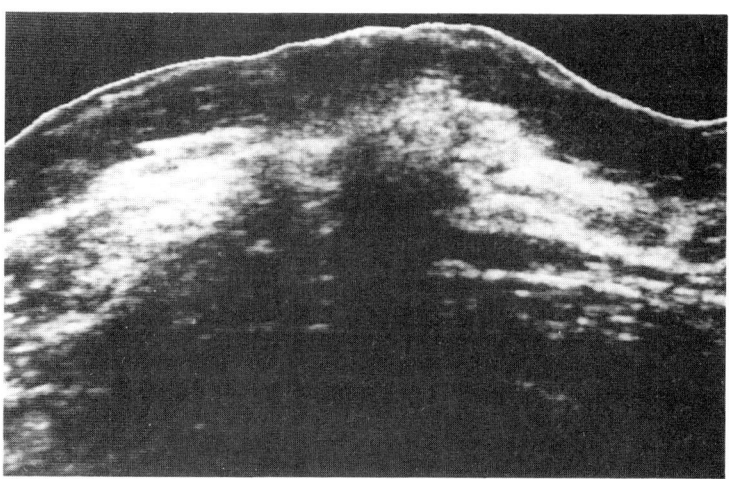

(b)

Figure 4 Radial scar: (a) X-ray showing a stellate shadow, with a suggestion of central fatty lucency; (b) ultrasound showing extensive attenuation suggesting carcinoma. Biopsy findings were a radial scar, with no malignancy

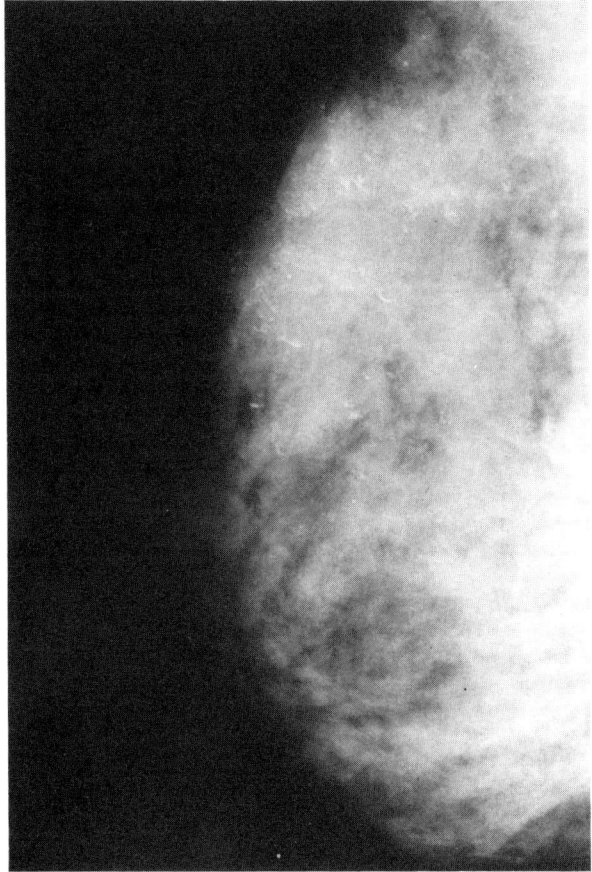

Figure 5 Sclerosing adenosis: X-ray showing segmental microcalcifications of varying morphology, possibly malignant. Biopsy showed sclerosing adenosis only

on occasions some suggestion of spiculation. Ultrasound has generally failed to show increased attenuation, a point which would be against a diagnosis of malignancy, although it is well recognized that some carcinomas fail to show this ultrasound sign[10]. In one patient, the diagnosis was made when fine needle aspiration produced slightly caseous-looking material containing foamy macrophages; further aspiration resolved the mass. We have been unable to find any report of these appearances in the literature.

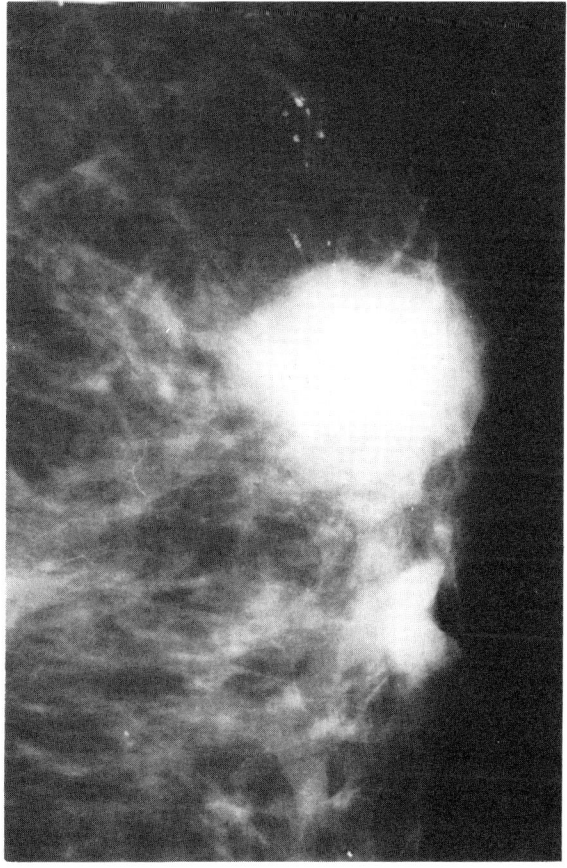

Figure 6 Duct ectasia: a round mass adjacent to the areola, with a suggestion of a few fine marginal striations, possibly carcinoma. Biopsy showed duct ectasia

CONCLUSION

Even with full preoperative evaluation, some benign processes cannot reliably be differentiated from malignancy, and excision biopsy will have to be considered for diagnosis. However, awareness of the overlapping features may lead to a watching policy rather than excision for some of these benign lesions.

REFERENCES

1. Forrest, P. (1986). *Breast Cancer Screening.* (London: Her Majesty's Stationery Office)
2. Guyer, P.B., Dewbury, K.C., Rubin, C.M., Royle, G.T. and Theaker, J. (1992). *Clin. Radiol.,* in press
3. Umpleby, H.C., Guyer, P.B., Moore, I., Royle, G.T. and Taylor, I. (1989). An evaluation of the pre-operative diagnosis and management of *Cystosarcoma phyllodes. Ann. R. Coll. Surg.,* **71**, 285–8
4. Nielsen, M., Jensen, J. and Anderson, J.A. (1985). An autopsy study of radial scar in the female breast. *Histopathology,* **9**, 287–95
5. Azzopardi, J.G. (1979). Problems in breast pathology. In Bennington, J.L. (ed.) *Major Problems in Pathology,* Vol. II, pp. 168–174. (London: W.B. Saunders)
6. Price, J.L., Thomas, B.A. and Gibbs, N.M. (1983). The Mammographic features of infiltrating epitheliosis. *Clin. Radiol.,* **34**, 433–5
7. Guyer, P.B. and Pearce, A. (1989). Characteristics of microcalcifications. *Br. J. Clin. Pract.,* **43**, Suppl. 68, 121–4
8. Tabar, L. and Dean, P.B. (1983). In Fronimhold, W. and Thurn, P. (eds.) *Teaching Atlas of Mammography,* pp. 119–29. (Stuttgart: George Thieme Verlag)
9. Lanyi, M. (1986). *Diagnosis and Differential Diagnosis of Breast Calcifications,* p. 86. (Berlin, New York, London, Paris: Springer Verlag)
10. Guyer, P.B. and Dewbury, K.C. (1987). *Sonomammography: An Atlas of Comparative Breast Ultrasound,* (Chichester, England: J. Wiley and Co.)

Index

227

effect on mammary tissue
  transplants 134
effect on epithelial proliferation
  137, 143, 147
role in menstrual cycle 106
oestrogen receptors
  and parity 145
  in natural menstrual cycle 144
  in oral contraceptive use 145
olfaction, role in menstrual cycle
  108
oncogene protein expression 153
oral contraceptive pill
  and breast cancer risk 139, 165
  and steroid receptors 145
  early use 169
  epidemiological studies 165
  latent effect 168
  long-term use 166
  use patterns 169
osteocalcin 81, 85
osteoporosis, and tamoxifen 185
ovarian cycle 103, 109
ovarian steroids 103
  action on stroma 117
ovulation 106

pain, *see under* mastalgia
papillary apocrine change 152
papillomata 204, 205
  intracystic 221
parity
  and breast cancer risk 68
  and contraceptive use 167
Patey, fistulotomy of 207
pectoral fasciitis 79
phyllodes tumours 217, 218
physiotherapy, use in lateral chest
  wall pain 77
pineal gland 106
pituitary–ovarian function 106

central nervous system and 107
plasma lipids as markers of breast
  cancer risk 67
potassium levels in breast cancer
  cyst fluid 177
progesterone
  effect on mammary tissue
    transplants 134
  effect on proliferation 132, 144
progesterone receptors
  and parity 145
  in natural menstrual cycle 144
  in oral contraceptive use 145
prolactin
  bioactivity and age 161
  bioassay 157
  levels in mastalgia 91
  problems with measurement 157
  radioimmunoassay 157
  role in breast cancer 157
prolactinoma 205
proliferation
  analysis of 153
  changes during menstrual cycle
    131, 143
  response to oestrogen alone 137
  response to progesterone 138
  time delay in response to
    oestrogen 147
proliferative breast disease 152
proteoglycans 116
psychological changes
  during menstrual cycle 111
  in women with benign breast
    disease 191

quality of life 191

radial scars
  comparison with malignancy 213
  management of 215, 222